Intuitive Eating

A Workbook That Works With Tips to Increase Your Health

(The Practical Guide to Develop Intuitive Eating)

Florence Poirier

Published By **Chris David**

Florence Poirier

Intuitive Eating: A Workbook That Works With Tips to Increase Your Health (The Practical Guide to Develop Intuitive Eating)

ISBN   978-1-77485-784-7

Legal & Disclaimer

TABLE OF CONTENTS

Chapter 1: The Disorders Of Eating Disorders

What is an eating disorder?

The term"eating disorder" is used to refer to the condition that is defined by an abnormal eating pattern and routines. These habits, result in severe changes and discomfort to the form and weight of the body. A large number of people are misinformed about eating disorders. to be a disease that is connected to lifestyle and food choices totally.

In addition to disrupting your everyday activities The illness can also affect your mental and emotional well-being. It could be times when you're being anxious over your diet or being embarrassed by your weight. This could lead you to withdraw from peoplefor the sake of expressing their worries about your health. The situation could result in depression as a supplementary manifestation.

The more time the condition persists and is not treated more, the greater the damage that occurs, for example, impacting digestion, bones, the skin, the strength of your gums and teeth, and even your heart's performance.

There are a variety of eating disorders which should not be dismissed lightly. They require care and expert aid. If you are aware of someone suffering from one of the eating disorders, you must urge the person to get medical attention and provide them with the emotional support they require. Additionally, you should know the symptoms and signs of these disorders to ensure you can determine if you are still in the health-related side or are on the brink of being affected by them.

Binge Eating

This causes people to eat huge amounts of food after one has experienced the sensation of having a full stomach. Many people who suffer from food cravings try to conceal it from their family and friends and are able to isolate themselves at times.

It is a similar eating disorder similar to Bulimia that is characterized by an adolescent loss of control over eating however, unlike Bulimia it does not have response to the loss of control. Every now and then, people overeat, and diagnosing this condition is difficult. But, if it happens more frequent and often but not necessarily due to the reason of hunger, it's an indication that something is not normal.

In the end, the majority of people suffering from binge eating disorders are overweight. They also run a higher likelihood of developing diseases related to the cardiovascular system. The majority of the time the eating disorders that are binge-like are usually associated with or preceded by low self-esteem and additionally, extreme emotions such as embarrassment, sadness and guilt. If it is not addressed properly this can further affect the progression of the disorder. The act of eating a lot is not necessarily harmful, but it becomes a problem when the person loses control of their eating.

In addition to emotion, there's a variety of food items that can trigger cravings. This is the case with carbohydrates. Foods that are high in carbohydrates and fats, according to researchers, stimulate the release of serotonin hormone that is found in the brain. This hormone results in pleasure-inducing feelings and emotions. The binge eaters are always inclined to favor these foods.

Signs associated with this disorder comprise:

* The tendency to overeat due to a lack of control

Feelings of guilt and shame following an overeating

* Binge eating, without any other

* Food intake that is higher than what was intended.

* Secret about overeating

Food Addiction

Certain people suffer from addiction to food. They are enthralled by certain kinds of food, and then give up. They're not able to quit even when they're full because they love the taste or taste. Food addicts and overeaters make use of food to feel a sense of satisfaction. They frequently try to break their eating habits however, as other addicts, they usually experience the possibility of return. Like addiction to alcohol and drugs the food addiction can be a problem with your daily life and cause stress in your relationship.

The majority of those who eat excessively or eat regularly suffer from stress-related disorders and have a negative body image. The stress they experience can stem from the condition itself. If you eat too much it is possible to feel guilty for what you did which can leave you feel stressed following the meal. If you're embarrassed by your actions, and try to conceal it from people around you and you are overwhelmed. Also, your issues with food cravings can cause you to be more likely to overeat. This can become a continuous cycle.

The people who are binge eaters also have a tendency to dislike how they appear. The negative image of their body makes them be compelled to cut down on their eating. Since they are always concerned about their appearance and how other people view about them, they are anxious. In addition, their constant anxiety of eating more food than they should make them feel even more stressed. These stress-related feelings lead them to eat more or nourish their bodies.

There are also those who give to themselves. They believe that they're already obese So why should try to alter their diet? They think it's impossible for them to lose weight and live a healthier lifestyle. Some do not bother to do anything because they believe that, in their mind they have their case sorted already.

Emotional eating

It's eating to meet the emotional desires. People tend to eat when they are feeling unhappy or stressed. They believe that if consume the food they long to eat during times of stress, they'll feel better. However, most times they experience a worse feeling since they guilt-ridden for eating more food than they ought to.

It is not healthy to eat emotionally. In addition to being a reason weight gain and causing anxiety, it does not allow you to deal with the root of the issue.

It's possible that you feel more relaxed while eating but after you've finished eating can it be said to guarantee that you'll never be overwhelmed ever again? It's true that feeling anxious or unhappy or sad occurs to everyone. I know that some people experience they are more often more than others. It's important to deal with stress in the correct way. You can try other ways to relax such as watching films and reading books. Or get help from a professional in how to manage stress. If you keep this unhealthy routine, it may cause weight gain even if you're not already there. It's never too late to make a change.

If you're feeling hungry emotionally you're likely to crave specific comfort food items. The majority of the time it's unhealthy foods like junk food, or high-calorie meals such as pizza and burgers.

You aren't able to be attentive and are not concerned with the food you consume and how it is prepared. You don't really relish eating You simply eat and eat and you'll take time to feel full since it's not your stomach which is full but your emotions.

Emotional hunger is a sudden sensation and sometimes inexplicably difficult to control. It is a sensation that you feel instantly and are then completely powerless to stop it. The majority of people give in to the craving immediately.

Most of us fail to recognize the connection between eating and our moods. Knowing what triggers us to engage with emotional food is the most important element to overcoming this harmful habit. The most common misconception we should disbelieve is that emotional eating being caused by negative emotions like anger, anxiety, stress or even grief. People do consume food when they are lonely, bored and sad, or stressed out or stressed out. However, we can all agree that at one time in our lives, we've been able to celebrate the good news by eating food. Children who were being given candy whenever they did something will keep doing this even after they reach adulthood. This is their method of rewarding their peers too. Positive feelings are a major factor in emotional eating. This is evident in Valentine day sweets and romantic treats as well as popcorn, and bags of chips while watching a film.

When it comes to eating emotional You must be aware that you're a human. That means you're an individual with a passion. You experience emotions like sadness, joy as well as anger and fear and many more. This leads to emotional eating. This means that you consume food according to the way you feel. In most cases individuals eat food to soothe themselves during times of devastation or grief. You must remove this habit and substitute it with something better.

For instance, if you're feeling low and you are feeling down, go to run. Being outside lets you get fresh air. Jogging is a great way to boost your heart rate as well as exercise your body. Both are great for you since they calm your body and can make you feel great. In addition they will keep you far from your fridge and keep you from looking for a tub of frozen ice cream. When you consume comfort food it is a good feeling initially. But eventually you realize that you regret what you did because you are aware you body health will be paying for it later.

In addition, you need to remove your negative and harmful nutrition-related beliefs. Don't be one of those who think food is the enemy. Food isn't your enemy. If you get fat this isn't the food's responsibility. It's your fault. If you hold these beliefs that you have, you'll develop an unhealthy relationship to food. This means that you have to modify your thinking about food.

Find the Triggers

Although it is generally acknowledged that emotional overeating can be triggered by emotion, there are other factors that act as triggers. Knowing your own triggers will significantly help you overcome emotional causes and symptoms of emotional eating

Emotional eating is the practice where someone consumes an excessive amount of food generally foods that are harmful like "junk food," so that they can feel more relaxed. In essence, those suffering who suffer from Emotional Eating Disorder make use of food to ease the stress or loneliness they're experiencing.

Be able to deal with your emotions

If your emotional issues aren't addressed in any manner, you'll carry through an emotional eating frenzies. Your positive emotions should find a way to express them. Find different ways to celebrate the occasion or milestone other than eating. Going bowling or going to the latest movie is a way to celebrate too. Beware of the popcorn unless you've prepared for it.

The idea of denying that your feelings are a problem isn't healthy, nor do you want to ignore your feelings. The fact that you ignore a problem doesn't mean it is not a problem. It's fine to express your emotions. You could be honest and say "I am angry at the moment." You could say, "I am depressed today." Be open about your feelings however, don't let them control you by consuming a lot of alcohol or screaming at people.

If your feelings are wildly out of hand, visiting an expert counselor could be beneficial. There are many people who have emotional issues requires counseling or therapy, however there's no reason not to seek this type of assistance when it is required. Anything that can help get your health back is what you should do if it is possible.

In certain societies, people haven't been taught to manage things that are difficult or difficult. Although this may be appealing however, it's not very beneficial. Children and adults alike are not taught to to experience and deal with the emotions that are unpleasant.

If you're angry accept the anger. Be aware of it, but don't let it spiral into a spiral that is out of control. If you're feeling depressed, you can go through the emotions But don't stay there. If you're depressed, you should allow yourself to feel the emotion, and then take it off your chest. Do you have a valid reason to be depressed, such as the loss of a loved one or a significant change in your life? If not, there could be a problem that requires medical attention. Mindfulness is not a way to avoid the emotions. It encourages you to confront the emotion and confront it.

If you're stressed take a look at the root of your stress. If you can remove something out of your life, then take it off your list. If the situation is one that you cannot leave and you need to come up with a plan to handle the issue. Counselors are an excellent source for these kinds of strategies.

However, in the meantime you should continue to do mindful eating to ensure the problem doesn't affect your eating habits more than it already does.

Overeating and under-eating

Over and under-eating can be a huge issue for many people. We are conditioned by society to believe that being thin can be the sole acceptable "norm" that leads many people to overeat and it is particularly a problem for women and girls in their teens.

This results in the phenomenon of under-eating because people are then prone to reduce certain foods , or even several foods, with their primary objective being to lose weight or keep the slim body weight they feel comfortable with.

However, we must keep in mind that we can't all appear alike (or be slim) since each individual has a unique body shape, bodies are different and our bodies' needs differ. So, you must make the best decision for you and to maintain your highest quality of life.

This is also true for eating too much since we be spending more of our time at work , and spend less time making healthy food. This means that fast food restaurants are earning more cash than ever before. Most people are inclined to buy fast food because it's the most easy and accessible option to take.

It is also where eating too much can be a problem, since individuals may be in the car or not eat meals often that leads to being over-indulged when they do manage to eat. It's extremely easy to overeat if one eats too quickly.

Although we're not suggesting that we should avoid eating any fast food however, the reality is that fast food isn't necessarily the healthiest food choice and, in fact, the consumption of too many fast foods can result in weight gain and health problems too.

It is essential to keep cooking and eating healthy , mindful meals and cut down on the fast-food habit to a conscious eating "treat" that we can enjoy looking at looking forward to. Consuming everything in moderation is essential to a being healthy and happy. Overeating is a frequent issue.

It is however simple to understand. Many people believe that they are overheated due to the weakness of their willpower. They think that they can't manage their appetites which is the reason they are unable to lose weight. In reality, they don't suffer from a lack of willpower. They are simply people who overeat and do not consume food when they eat. What is this referring to?

If you don't take a bite when eating it is not the case that you are fully present throughout your meal. You're not conscious of the flavor or how it is nourishing your body. Your brain is missing out on an essential aspect of your nutrition, one that involves satisfaction and tasting. Your brain may believe that you didn't consume enough food or did not eat anything at all. Then, you believe that you're hungry and take in more calories than you're supposed to. If you are trying to avoid overindulging, make sure that you keep your attention and alertness during meals.

There is also this belief that when eating fast it boosts your metabolism. It is actually true that eating slowly can increase your metabolism. If you eat quickly you stress your body. Remember that we are not designed biologically for eating at high speeds. If you consume food quickly it puts your body in a state of physiologic stress. This results in less digestion, nutrient assimilation and burning of calories. In turn, it increases appetite and excretion of nutrients.

As your metabolism slows down, it will increase the efficiency of your nutrition. Additionally, you can taste food more and this increases your enjoyment. It is important to improve your eating pleasure to be more satisfied with it. There is no need to consume more food. Just be aware of its flavor, presentation as well as overall high-quality. It triggers a feeling of relaxation in addition to aids digestion and assimilation. Furthermore, you'll have the opportunity to chew your food more attentively. You can be sure you are able to digest it correctly.

Anorexia Nervosa

Anorexia is a psychological well-being disorder as. The sufferers are constantly distracted from food and self-perception. They don't eat or count calories to much or eat very small amounts to maintain their health. Even if they aren't often, they feel anxious about the belief that they're overweight, and are constantly trying to lose weight. Although the disorder is more prevalent for young women but it is now recognized to be affecting the younger generation of men and women than previously believed. Studies show that anorexia typically starts between 13 and 30 years of age.

The signs include weight loss, not eating enough food to maintain an ideal weight, a incorrect perception of one's appearance and worry about increasing weight and becoming overweight. The patient may begin to subject himself or herself to extreme diets that result in rapid weight loss. However, many patients refuse to eat, even though their weight is lower than the normal. Due to a misperception of their appearance, they believe that they're not slim as they ought to be and keep on a diet. Their fear of becoming overweight drives them to over workouts, the use drugs to help them lose weight and consume less food. As time passes, this pattern takes on the characteristics of fixation , and frequently reaches the point of being at risk of becoming suffering from starvation.

Although they aren't necessarily related to anorexia, here we do present some of the symptoms that can be seen in the case of anorexia.

Mental Signs

* Mental fixation on eating and one's weight

A deformed perception of one's look

* Self-esteem is defined by appearance and weight

Self-judgment and a desire for perfection

Psychological indicators

* Clinical depression

* A low view of self-worth

* Changes in mood

Social Signs

* Do not make contact with your friends.

* Worsening relationship with family

* Productivity and engagement in work or assessment is facing significant decrease (however due to perfectionist tendencies, it's not always the case)

Behavioural Signs

* Training or exercise that is too intense

* Refusal of eating and obsessiveness about calories intake

* Hidden behavior regarding the food and weight

• Self-harm and tendencies to suicide, frequent use of substances

For men, anorexia typically occurs in conjunction with mental health issues and usually follows a that they've been overweight. Anorexic males often have a negative perception of how they appear.

For women, the symptoms of anorexia are ascribed to a general feeling of discontentment with their body, and a desire for being as slim as they can. Female anorexics typically exhibit patterns of excessive perfectionist.

In addition to the mental signs the physical manifestations of anorexia for those who are young are connected to their development and growth. People's lives are severely affected. Their interest in the activities they used to take pleasure in is evidently diminished. Many sufferers exhibit symptoms of depression in clinical cases.

While anorexia can be described by the term "lack of appetite" people who suffer from anorexia tend not to lose appetite. They love eating and have a feeling of hunger however they don't think about eating as other people do as can be observed in a myriad of different behavior patterns. To give a few examples that they may be lie about their food intake and presenting excuses for not wanting to eat, saying they've already eaten but they haven't, hiding the amount of weight they've actually shed and so on.

If malnutrition or the threat of starvation have begun to impact your body, medical steps should be taken. Doctors treat illnesses that result from anorexia nervosa , such as osteoporosis, heart disease as well as clinical depression. When you are beginning to heal, a physician will continue to monitor your health and ensure that you stay in the weight you are healthy.

Bulimia Nervosa

The eating disorder known as bulimia can be that is characterized through frequent bouts of excessive eating that are immediately followed by vomiting, usage of diuretics and the use of enemas or purgatives. Most of the time, those suffering from bulimia are able to conceal their behaviors because they are ashamed of their excessive eating. They are aware that their eating habits aren't normal. It's a dangerous condition because the symptoms of the disorder aren't immediately apparent and the diagnosis is difficult to establish.

They don't always suffer from weight problems. Sometimes, they are normal weight. The obsession to shed weight, caused by emotional or mental issues does not allow them to control of their bulimic attacks. If they consume the identical amount of food they consume the previous day, their bodies suffer from malnutrition that can result in a significant loss of weight, but this doesn't always happen.

Bulimia nervosa is most prevalent in women aged between 15 and 30. The final stage of bulimia nervosa can be the manifestation of severe clinical depression, which could cause the sufferer to commit suicide.

There are many ways to lose weight , by putting yourself to extreme diets. Bulimia's weight is normal, but can go up to five pounds heavier or lighter in the midst of an eating spree and times of fasting. Bulimia nervosa sufferers tend to be anxious and depressed, or exhibit mood changes. Bulimia is a common occurrence of cases is associated with anorexia. It is difficult to determine which one is most prevalent.

There are several indicators to help you in identifying those who may have developed the disorder known as bulimia nervosa

* Bad teeth due to acidity of the stomach when vomiting

* Using the toilet after eating (to be able to eliminate);

* Hands that are injured caused by being forced into the throat to cause vomiting;

* Fatigue, weakness or fainting

* Dehydration;

* Heart-related heart malfunctions;

* Tongue and throat sores;

* Disorders or disturbances that disrupt the menstrual cycle

• Often, eating too much, especially food items that cause weight gain;

Bulimia nervosa and its treatment

1. Understand the nature of the issue.

• Discuss the subject with someone else, and don't expect them to make a judgement.

Beware of people who are only able to talk about diets and food.

It is important to realize that you are able to be in control of what you consume.

* Get the assistance by a professional or talk about it with an expert psychologist.

* Seek advice regarding the illness.

Be aware that you are healthy in your weight especially when you feel the need to eliminate of foods you've eaten.

* Develop a plan to manage emotional difficulties and depression.

* Find positive role models that you can identify with and help you in boosting your self-esteem. Be aware that mass media projections of skinny models, or even actors typically reflect unhealthy lifestyles.

Establish a routine eating pattern and avoid exposing yourself to diets.

Chapter 2: The Benefits Of Intuitive Eating

It's obvious that you appear good looking when you're healthy, that is the state that which intuitive eating can help you attain however, that's not the only thing you will appreciate. When you are in the habit of eating intuitively and make it your daily routine you will reap the many advantages that you can reap. But, before getting there, it's crucial to be aware of how to differentiate the real hunger from the cravings.

How to distinguish real hunger from Cravings

It is likely that you have eating habits that make you reach for food when you're bored or apathetic It is also possible that you consume a lot of food when you're annoyed by people or are upset over something. These, in fact are not good reasons to be eating. And because you're so used to eating food in this way, you could be unable to discern whether your desire to eat stems from the physical needs of your body, or for other motives that are not related to your body.

* If you feel embarrassed every time you eat it is likely that you're reaching for food even though you're not really hungry.

If you are eating fast and aren't able to find the time to chew, it is likely that your body's not the one that is demanding to be fed.

If you've had the feeling of eating in stressful situations it is likely that there is an emotional urge that is seeking to be met, disguised as hunger.

* If you've noticed that you're eating more often, even after having consumed a substantial meal, the odds are the food you're eating isn't for the good of your body.

* If, after eating you feel stuffed then it's likely that you've consumed more than your body needs or perhaps you ate even though you weren't really hungry, in the literal sense.

* If you feel you're hungry and your first impulse is to go to the store for some nuts, vegetables or fruits, then you are likely to be feeling genuine hunger. In contrast when you think you're hungry, and the first thought that comes to your mind is

chocolate, ice cream or doughnuts You are most likely simply bored or in search to feel some sort of consolation. These foods are usually a way to fulfill cravings and, no matter the amount you consume, the feeling of hunger isn't likely to go away.

Once you've come to comprehend the body's language and become accustomed to responding to it in a manner that is appropriate eating with ease will be an integral part of your daily life. Through this process, you'll benefit from:

(1)Enhanced digestion

The main points to be aware of when it comes to intuitive eating are concerned are:

(i)The need to eat only when you truly hungry

(ii)The necessity of eating food until your hunger is gone or until you're satisfied. It is not recommended to eat until you are full.

So long as you're paying attention to these two essential aspects that your digestive system won't be overwhelmed by the amount of salt, fat, and sugar it has a hard time processing and eliminate.

One of the most afflicted that you infuse you body, or continue eating for a long time is your liver, as it must continue to work to remove toxins from these food items and also to process the fat. Naturally, your stomach is also on an overdrivebecause each food you eat that you eat, it needs to produce more enzymes and acids to treat it. When you've mastered the art of mindful eating the body gets enough time to relax until the next real craving strikes.

Intuitive eating helps you avoid digestive issues that result from putting freshly consumed food on partially digested foods. If you expose your digestion system this situation, it is confused about which stage of digestion it should subject to the food. It is no wonder that people who eat in a hurry and without any thought of hunger are constantly complaining of constipation, stomach indigestion, and other digestive issues.

(2)Reduced instances of stress

It is known that intuitive eaters don't have as much stress in their lives when they make an effort to lose weight and diet. weight. Because of the freedom that intuitive eaters enjoy , and the ease of being under pressure about the amount, what and the best time to eat, they tend to be happy and free of anxiety. They tend to be more emotionally healthy than those who tend to suffer from depression and anxiety. Actually, a large portion of people in this group are constantly in self-deflection, and this can hurt their chances of success with their diet program.

However the opposite is true. When these people who are dieting switch to intuitive eating more often, they're less anxious and stressed, and in a short time their psychological well-being improves. There are many reasons dieters feel stressed compared to those who eat intuitively however one of the most important is that they are able to unwind and enjoy the mealinstead of focusing on the ingredients of food items and their quantity of calories. Each time you remind you to stop reaching for the food item solely to combat weight gain, it's the perfect way to create stress. Without any conditions, you're content that your body no longer needs what you've been vowing not to consume as there isn't anything as such, in any case.

(3)Reduction or stabilization the weight

As an sensitive eater, you are in no fear of failure, since you don't have a predetermined goal in your diet. Therefore, there is nothing to feel disappointed about every day. You have instead allowed your body to decide what it requires, and you nourish it according to. However, if you decide on a specific amount of food items for breakfast or lunch for example, and the demands of your body will likely vary daily and night, is it not likely that you'll end up overfilling your body at times, while eating it to death in other instances?

Since in intuitive eating, you pay attention to your body's needs and give it only what is required and you end with settling at a perfect weight. It's been proven that those who practice intuitive eating have higher BMIs.

Additionally, there is the possibility of eating intuitively being the reason for a relaxed environment as well as direct diets that cause the increase in stress levels. Biochemically, it is known that cortisol, a hormone associated with stress is also the reason for weight increase. The bottom line is that people who are on weight loss programs risk jeopardizing their odds of success due to the stress-inducing environment they are in.

(4)Strengthening self-esteem

There aren't many things as difficult as setting a goal that you set for yourself, like you do with weight loss, and failing disastrously. Of course, thinking about it could cause anxiety. Every when you consider failing, you consider eating less. If you're having a less nutritious diet even though your body really needs more. What impression do you imagine you'll be sending to it? Your body will perceive you as indicating that there is a shortage of food, so it is better to not use everything you've given it before.

Do you realize how this can hinder your efforts in losing weight? The body slows down its metabolism and stores up calories it should would have burned, and when you are gaining weight despite all your efforts to eat smaller you feel angry and feel as a failed. This is why your self-esteem declines and you're in a difficult emotional position. What can people who are suffering emotionally? They look for comfort foods, and other bad routines. What happens when you are eating what you want such as with intuitive eating yet you are losing pounds that are unhealthy? Your self-esteem increases as you are a more content person, and might even meet more people. Positive people who have an optimistic outlook on life are attracted by similar people. In the world of social interaction this is the way"the law of attraction" operates.

(5)Enhanced body awareness

When you are used to eating intuitively the body will become automatic. You can even detect in your body's signs that it's deficient in, say iron, and you will be in a position of resolving the problem without having to consult a doctor to undergo more complex and costly procedures.

In essence, when you're intuitive eating, you don't just read your body's signals of satiety and hunger, but you also look at its signals in the whole. That's why you are able to respond to each of them with the most pertinent way, unlike instances where people use food to ward off signs unrelated to hunger. Intelligent eaters aren't likely serve an entire meal because they are tired after having a restful day. They will likely realize that the food they've had for a while is deficient in vegetables and other iron-rich foods and, in order to rectify this, they'll to respond with plenty of salads made from vegetables. The body will long for these foods and won't allow you to go to the butchery or meat shop without a piece of liver.

This is an advantage that traditional dieters don't have because they aren't focused in listening to the signals of their body. This is why losing weight isn't always the same as healthy living. You could take the exact same calories as an intuitive eating style and feel tired, while the person who is intuitive is always active due to heeding the body's signals to eat the right food. When you are an intuition-driven eater, term calories is not mentioned anywhere. It's all about what does it feel like?

Chapter 3: Emotional Hunger Versus Physical Hunger

From the time we were infants We have been taught to recognize food as the necessity to eat. Food is a necessity. Food is what ensures that we are alive. The nutrients that we get from food replenish our damaged tissues. We are familiar with the fundamentals of how our digestive system functions. We were taught that we should take three meals in the day to fuel ourselves. However, that's nowhere far from the reality. Our ancestors did not eat three meals in a day. Our bodies weren't made to eat three meals a day.

It's getting worse because there's so much junk food that is available for purchase. There are at least one or two fast food outlets just around the corner. Our society has been eating a lot! We're always chasing one or the other. It's nuts!

This is why I am now to explain the difference between REAL physical hunger or emotional, hunger. It's because it's only when you know the difference you'll be better able to take care of yourself the next time you're contemplating going to the Taco Bell again.

Physical Hunger

The true physical hunger occurs the moment when your body demands food. It's undeniable. The stomach feels like a black hole that is empty. You may feel a bit lightheaded or dizzy. Sometimes you get nauseous. It's difficult to concentrate on what you're doing. You are easily annoyed such as, "Why does the air smell like air? What's up with that?"

When you feel hungry, that you must take a bite, and the quicker you eat the better. That is why physically hungry is something that you can notice. There are physical manifestations. It's not in your head.

All of this is enabled through a hormone called Ghrelin. Ghrelin is produced from the stomach, brain pancreas, brain, and small intestinal tract. It is responsible for a variety of things within the body of a human, at present we're focused on its role to act as "hunger hormone."

Ghrelin is the brain's signal to must get your pie hole open and pour pie into it. It boosts the appetite of a person and absorption of food and is the main reason for the storage of fat in humans.

If we're deficient in energy in our body the body produces ghrelin inside the stomach walls and it then sends out an electrical signal to the brain that increases the appetite and intake of food. It also plays a significant part in the body's mass.

Ghrelin is an arch-nemesis known as leptin. You didn't know there was all the drama within your body, wouldn't you? Leptin is contrary to the effects of ghrelin. What's that? You've guessed it. It can reduce appetite. Thin people are believed to have lower levels of ghrelin , and also higher levels of leptin and the opposite is the case with overweight people.

These are the fundamentals of hunger physical. If your stomach starts to rumble, be aware that there's an urgent situation!

Emotional Hunger

The feeling of hunger is in your head. You may feel that you're experiencing a hunger inside that no other food will satisfy. It is possible that the issue is an emotional hunger. It's a fairly frequent occurrence. Whatever the case, emotional hunger can be a challenge to conquer, especially if you've been consuming it in such a way that you can't stop eating in a way that is automatic. However, you can defeat it! The mind is the best matters!

On Emotions

It's normal for us for us to experience emotions. This is a large aspect of what we do as human beings. The emotions are important and crucial. You should be as attentive to them as you do the food you consume or the job you perform.

It is for this reason that we need to be aware of our eating habits and what causes us to become dependent on comfort food. When you're capable of addressing your issues, you need to give yourself an honest assessment. As a human being, you possess a level of intelligence that is unmatched. This level of intelligence allows you to think critically and solve problems. What good is intelligence without emotion? Even Siri is emotional! The emotions prevent us from becoming completely robotic with necessary attributes such as empathy affection, compassion, love and more.

Whatever the reason you be suffering emotionally; you can channel your positive energy on getting better. It might take longer than you would like. But you'll surely be better.

Emotional Hunger Triggers

It is simple to spot if know the signs you're seeking. Have you ever been informed by a relative or lover that you're too intimate? You call too much? You've tried not to but you are unable to get rid of yourself. These are the signs that you're seeking emotional security. Afraid to be alone.

When you behave like this when you behave this way, you're more likely to interpret meanings that aren't there. It is difficult to feel hurt when someone doesn't behave in the way you would like to be acting or the way you imagined their reactions. If things don't turn out the way you had planned you experience an emotional decline that leads you to eat more emotionally to satisfy your emotional craving.

Since it's as if eating food can be the sole thing in your life that isn't judging you.

It doesn't have to be that way!

Overthinking

People who are emotionally hungry think that they have the inside of everyone's heads, that they are aware of the thoughts of everyone and what they are commenting on them. Aiming to gain acceptance and attention solely based on of the conclusions you've been able to make is an invitation to catastrophe. Why? If you're upset, your emotional stomach gets triggered and the then, before you know it you're at three-quarters full of one litre of Ben Jerry's.

A major characteristic of people who are emotionally hungry is the desire to adhere to certain beliefs or behaviours that are accepted by a certain group of people in order not to be left out or hung.

Self-Loathing and dissatisfaction

The majority of the time people who are emotionally hungry try to appear, behave and talk like others. Most often, they are people of high social standing. They are looking to achieve the things that the emotionally hungry individual has failed to achieve. Many admiring fans, friends and a beautiful figure six pounds and muscles and a great job and a remarkable ability to stay on diets, etc.

People who are emotionally hungry are frequently heard saying "How I would love to be like this woman and not have to control what she eats"

"How I'd love to appear like that! I would be able to wear anything would like!" The more they dream to be happy, the more depressed they become and the weaker their resolve grows as well as the greater amount they snack emotionally.

The entire concept behind emotional hunger is the desire to experience something that is distinct from the usual boring things. The desire in order to "feel awake."

Methods for People to Deal With Emotional Hunger

When some people eat to cope with their feelings while others participate in more sporting activities to feel more alive and, in turn, fills them with emotional satisfaction. This is an excellent thing!

For those who want intimacy with others, they can have sexual contact - but not necessarily to connect with another person however, but to experience whatever it is they desire to feel. For the majority of people, sexual intimacy is a normal part of life. Someone who is hungry for emotional satisfaction might consider it more than just a way to have fun, however. For them, casual sexual activity is a type that is a form of "nourishment." They stay clear of emotional turmoil that makes them appear inadequate emotionally and instead go on for thrills. They are trying to believe that they are adequate.

It's not the fault of anyone else! In a society that is purely judging that a person cannot be fit enough and slim, attractive enough, or simply attractive enough, they are feeling like they don't belong anyplace. Sex seems like the most convenient method of convincing ourselves that we've had our desire for pleasure satisfied.

It's not enough.

After a certain period, it isn't working as well or appears to not work in the same way it did in the past. We feel as if we're getting approval from that person we're interacting with. We believe that we are adequate. We believe that no one else's opinions matter. We believe that we are worthy of someone else's attention , and this is accompanied by "feel great" hormones released by the brain following sex. We feel satisfied in the moment, and any other individual's opinion is not important since you feel "good."

If you're able connect, then the odds are that you're prone to having more sexual friends than is healthy. Don't forget that there are plenty of STDs in the world to get you into hot water at some point or another.

Sex and emotional pain

Although studies have shown that sexual activity can ease the sorrow, sadness, or the anger that one experiences towards things, it's not an all-time solution to the root cause. While it is possible to look into your sexuality a healthy way but you shouldn't be using it to deal with unwholesome emotions. This is, unfortunately, the way that most people do. Studies show that the majority of those who are involved in casual and random sexual activity are feeding an emotional craving. In an effort to prove they're worthy of being.

If you don't think you're able to overcome emotional hunger by yourself It is possible to look for a trusted friend or a friend. If, in spite of the assistance systems at your disposal, getting through this is a challenge, don't be ashamed or nervous to seek help from a professional.

Emotional and drug-related hunger and drugs

Like sex, people are prone to use drugs as a way to cope with anxiety. It is common among those who want to alleviate their hurt. It could be the grief of losing someone, the hurt of a broken home , or physical pain.

There are many temporary solutions that people can use to help them figure out what to do to satisfy their emotional craving. Some of them are self-destructive such as drug use and alcohol. Some people are uncomfortable in social settings, which is why they prefer to stay in a secluded area and adjust to their personal environment rather than interact with others , and risk being treated unfairly.

If you feel as if you've lost control of your life. If you are unable to manage the consumption of certain substances or if you realize that you're making use of these substances solely to satisfy your needs for emotional satisfaction It is recommended to seek out help from a therapist or a doctor.

To the most emotional people who are emotionally hungry, the thought of being separated or in relationships can be terrifying. To get rid of or reduce the feeling of loneliness you'll likely do things that are not healthy for your well-being. What you do can fill the gap in your emotional void that you're so afraid of.

The emotional hunger is triggered by breakups

The most emotionally hungry people who are in relationships respond negatively to the thought of breaking up. They don't feel that there's an issue and often don't believe they're the reason for the issue. People with these issues have a difficult to accept rejection.

Because people who are emotionally hungry tend to want to be accepted and have a connection to other people, they typically don't know how to behave in a respectful manner, as they have a difficult time doing it.

The battle against emotional hunger is all about working on your brain, and reprogramming yourself to manage problems in a more positive way. Make sure you have friends who are willing to put as much effort into your relationships as you are.

So, we've discovered that hunger for emotional reasons doesn't have to require constant emotional eating however it could develop into it when other ways of coping don't work for you.

Let's now tackle this head-on.

Chapter 4: Distracting Yourself

Alternatives to eating that distract you from the food

Recognizing that the urge to eat in a manner which is not in line with the diet you have planned is your brain's primitive voice communicating its survival instincts but then choosing to ignore it, will require you to refrain from eating out of emotion.

If that's all you do, you could be stuck in a never-ending loop in which you are compelled to eat, but you realize that it's your brain's primitive part and not you that is begging to eat. You can ignore the urge to eat repeated again.

There is no food this way, which is great but it's not the most enjoyable way to pass the time . If it's all you do, it's possible that you'll get tired of it and will eventually eat some food to keep it quiet.

To avoid the unfortunate circumstance you have the option of choosing, after you have heard you were hearing the voice from your brain's primitive part and decided to ignore it, take a break and engage in a different thing to do other than eating, and achieve some peace.

All of us know how it is when we are so involved in something that we fail to take our food in. We skip a meal, or two, or even more, and don't even realize that we're hungry.

Engaging in distractions, when we are tempted to indulge in emotional eating, operates with the same principles. We lose track of eating when we're distracted by something enough captivating to keep our focus.

The secret to avoiding distractions is that they are effortless and simple to carry out. They should be accessible without any effort or energy and be activities that you like or can be considered to be acceptable.

It is also important to choose things that you do because of habit, and not necessarily the new things you try very rarely, or choose to do because you think you ought to.

It's permissible to keep yourself entertained by engaging in a novel if that's something you regularly do as a way to escape or distract yourself. But don't keep yourself entertained with War and Peace, or Moby Dick, if you do not normally read novels.

Important note is to be cautious about engaging in an activity that you do when eating. If, for instance, you find yourself slouching away watching TV with cookies on the table watching TV may not be a good choice for you.

If you don't see a alternative in the list below that you do not think of as eating and you are unable to find other similar activities which don't require food, then seek out alternatives that are soothing instead.

However, it is likely that you'll be able to choose a distraction isn't associated with eating.

Be aware that these distractions are a fallback option for those times those who don't have the desire to take on more beneficial activities.

There's no reason to utilize them, however, allow yourself to use them when you aren't able to muster the courage or desire to make use of the alternatives later on.

There's a high chance that you'll no longer require to be distracted by thoughts of food after you've learned how to utilize EEESY(tm) to calm and calm your brain's primitive part and, as you progress through the process, you most likely will not.

However, in the meantime, allow yourself the right to relax when you're able to accomplish.

Activities to distract

1. Television watching. This is the top item on the list because for many it is a perfect fit for all the criteria mentioned above. It's not difficult and is easily accessible, and is something we often use to keep our minds off of things.

It's totally uninvolved, and it can be very enjoyable , particularly when you have a wide selection of entertainment options that are accessible.

We often associate TV watching with eating, here's an method that could assist you in resisting cravings for food when watching TV Watch something that's not compatible with eating, or something that can keep you from eating like a scary film or a documentary about diseases. It's also helpful to watch something that doesn't have commercials, which typically promote food.

If this is an thing that appeals to you it's best to make sure you have a program that you enjoy.

If you're looking for some distractions while watching television -- and it's likely to happen, pick one of the other options on the options.

2. Reading. There's nothing so dreadful as a sloppy novel in the event that it transports readers to a world that is far removed from the worries and anxieties of the real one.

There's nothing worse to be a part of than reading an e-book about romance in the evening on a Fridayand when you're exhausted from a hectic working week to accomplish any task that requires more effortand you're escaping to books rather than eating.

3. Playing video games. It's possible that you don't have an everyday Halo night however if you like playing video games, there's nothing wrong with them being distracting.

4. Internet activities. This might include surfing on the Internet and taking part in virtual worlds like

Second Life, engaging in online forums, and many other online activities.

It's true that you're wasting your time but when you're not eating your meals while browsing, it can be a compelling and useful divert from food.

Chapter 5: Tips To Be Successful In Intuitive

Eating And Avoid Common Errors

Are you ready to start your journey towards intuitive eating? It's easy however it takes some time to adjust to your body's needs and preferences. Make a list of goals for yourself Learn to understand the body's signals and communicate. Examine your schedule to ensure you have sufficient time in the day to eat when you are hungry, and make time for relaxation, exercise and meditation. This section will concentrate on the common mistakes and errors that could hinder your progress towards maintaining an optimal health and wellness through mindful eating.

Avoid Skipping Meals

This is an excellent suggestion to anyone. It's not always a good idea to skip meals particularly if your schedule doesn't permit enough time for a break. If you are expecting this to happen and plan ahead, wake up early in order to get breakfast ready. Take note of the levels of hunger in the morning to decide how much to consume. Consider bringing a small snack at work or to school just in case you have an chance to satisfy your appetite when you feel that you have to delay or skip lunch. If you are eating small or large portions be sure to have food that is nutritious and tasty just in the event of. Even the most well-planned schedules may be altered at any time and being prepared will reduce anxiety.

Do not drink enough water

Hunger is a sign of dehydration. If you are feeling hungry, drink plenty of water first. Hydration is among the most effective methods to maintain your health. It also helps regulate your appetite signals, to ensure that when you feel the urge to eating, it's an expression of hunger and not because of other reasons. If drinking water throughout the day isn't appealing to you, you can try adding lime, lemon or cucumber. Sparkling water is an alternative. Herbal teas are fantastic in colder weather, to make sure you're hydrated. Fruits are packed with water and sugar that is naturally occurring and can give you an energy boost between meals when needed. It is okay to drink coffee when consumed in moderation. However, it is best to avoid drinking water with coffee because it could have the effect of dehydrating.

Setting unrealistic goals

A lot of us have goals for our diets but, often they aren't achievable. The media, ads and diet plans promote quick fixes and certain methods to shed weight quickly however, it's only useful for a short period of time. In the most extreme instances, when weight loss is required due to health reasons an expert in medicine or nutritionist might offer a specific set of guidelines for eating. However, even within this framework it is possible to mindfully eat and be practicedby paying attention to the way food affects you and the time you consume food. Making healthy choices could be detrimental in the event that we eat food when we're not hungry , or eat excessively when we're in a state of mind and not paying attention to our body's signals.

Set your sights on one thing at each time, if it is necessary to avoid disappointment and disappointment. Also don't expect to lose many pounds or reduce anxiety levels and reduce your sugar levels at once. However, if you're eating a healthy diet and exercise regularly, even at a moderate level, you'll be seeing positive results in some weeks. It's not necessary to believe that overnight changes will happen and then can be shared on social media and get to receive a scathing reaction. The most effective individuals in losing 100 pounds or becoming more athletic and fit, have to dedicate many months, or even years, in order to reach their goals. Once the goal has been achieved however, maintenance is still required and should be continued. The practice of mindfulness can help you to understand the importance of maintenance right from the beginning, so that it is an everyday part of life.

Obstacles to intuitive eating The Emotional Response to Food and the Changing habits

There are habits we all have which are difficult to change or break and isn't something that you can change in a single day. Recognizing that a bad habit can be the beginning of making improvements, since it indicates that we are aware of the problem. Habits that form are often formed due to an event other than our own life. For instance, we might indulge in eating when we're in a state of emotional distress or to relax after a difficult event. It is common when people are grieving or experiencing an overwhelming sense of loss. Food may be used to mask the loss to help cope. If you're experiencing difficulties It is essential not to blame yourself, specifically for the way you eat. Recognize that it's temporary, and eventually when you're at a point of readiness, you can modify your way of thinking about food. The key is being aware. An effective method is meditation that allows you time to reflect without judgement, and to set achievable goals.

Avoid multi-tasking when eating

Making a deadline, talking on the internet or in person working on a project are all things people do at meals. It is most common in the lunch break, whether as an alternative to a "working break" in a method to reduce time and ease the pressure of trying to finish the work work that was started after lunch, although the opposite can happen. If you are trying to balance both of these tasks the way you eat and your body's signals can be disrupted. This causes a disconnect between food items and. This is the time that you could feel stressed to get back to work after lunch, or even in an informal and social setting, lose that feeling that you get when you enjoy eating your meal in peace and free of distraction. If you're strapped to time, allowing an adequate amount of time to savor your meal is a good idea to begin. Set down your computer files and quit the computer and walk in a tranquil and peaceful area. Food, however you decide to eat them, and if you have enough time and space are the best time to be at the center of your life and other activities are put off until you're done.

If you like eating with your coworkers, family members and your others, make it an enjoyable occasion. Be positive and have fun. If lunch at work is what you wish to accomplish, look for pleasure in your food whenever you are able to chew and take in every bite. Limit your multitasking in order to maintain a steady pace in your break. Your colleagues may notice that you eat slower and relish the flavor the food. It might be appropriate to discuss the food you eat and be grateful for what you've got. This can help other people observe the way you approach food intuitively and can motivate them to do the same!

What is emotional eating? How do you recognize and cope with Emotional Eating Behaviors

Emotional eating can be defined as an emotional response to food as a way to cope with stressful situations and stress in daily life. It can be a habitual behavior as a way to fill a need or gap in our lives which we are struggling with. In certain situations, when it becomes repeated and severe, eating disorders could occur. Most people see it as an indication of responding to anxiety, sadness or other emotional issues through food, even when there isn't any hunger. This can lead to an eating pattern that is characterized by binge eating or eating too much and, in some instances the inability to eat for a time until the hunger pangs are unbearableand cause people to overeat. In extreme instances, bulimia and anorexia are two examples of eating disorders that force people to avoid eating (anorexia) or flit in between having too many food items and then requiring you to stop eating food intake and shed pounds (bulimia).

Food can be more than just food. It's reward, means of coping or the source of comfort. The phrase "comfort food" refers to the need to eat food in order to get through a difficult situation like the breakup of a relationship and losing work or feeling of being a failure when expectations aren't met. It's not a good idea in the long run but it does make people feel better immediately. Films and TV shows occasionally show characters chomping on an ice cream tub following the breakup of their spouse. This is a response to a stressful event.

As we get older, we are taught to link food to various aspects of our lives. A lollipop, or an ice-cream cone is a reward for good behavior , or an additional slice of cake in exchange for doing chores. It could also be restricting, or even punitive in the event that portions or kinds of food are restricted if you were pressured to lose weight and consume food in a particular manner. There could be good intentions for both, but ultimately children learn to view food as a means to punish, reward or to provide. It's not an easy thing to change, but it is possible to do so by

59

acknowledging the ways in which these characteristics are ingrained in our minds at an early age, and understanding the reaction toward food when we encounter some of these issues in our adulthood:

As an adult, a reward might be to have an extra slice of cake in order to reward healthy eating habits in one week into a new diet

The punishment could be a restriction on your food choices during the month to for example, to "correct" the effects of a binge, or period of time when you indulged in foods that are considered to be forbidden through a diet

The choice to eat food is to deal with grief over loss, frustration or stress from events in our lives

What's the first sign that you are suffering from emotional eating? Cravings! They are not uncommon and we are all too familiar with them. They can occur even when you're not hungry, and are in response to an incident. For instance, if you find yourself overwhelmed in your job, you could want chocolate or even a bag of chips. The flavor could be attractive and so is the texture or flavor.

It might seem unrelated initially, to satisfy your cravings by eating a tiny piece of chocolate, but since the stress response is a food-related one the craving will persist and develop into a habit. The first time you taste the milk chocolate after dealing with an uneasy client at work might be euphoric, and later you'll crave another, then another. It's a pattern that develops, which is a connection between your mood and your food. Your portions could also increase while you try to ease your anxieties However, at the end, there's no way out, and your eating habits are difficult to keep.

How can you stay clear of the traps of eating out for emotional reasons? Be aware of your mood before you head for your next meal. Are you at home, In your home, work or at an event at a place that gives you an uneasy feeling? In the first place, figure out whether you're actually hungry by using the scale ranging from one and 10. If you score your hunger higher than 10 it could be beneficial to consume food, however, ensure that you're in an area that is calm and unhurried before you start your meal. If you are feeling hungry, it's the perfect moment to eat, but with as low a pressure and emotional stress as is possible. If you're working in a crowded area, locate a space to relax and unwind. Do some deep breathing exercises and choose the best place to eat your meal.

If you find yourself craving food, think about what you feel. Are you sad, angry or overwhelmed? If you're feeling emotional rage or mood of anger, put from eating until you have brought yourself to a calm place and away from the surroundings which can contribute to these feelings. It's likely to take less time than you think , and it could be as simple to leave the office or work area and going outside to walk around an area park. If that isn't offered, then choose a tranquil space in your office with no distractions. Sometimes , this is difficult to locate if your workplace is crowded and chaotic. Just a few minutes in a bathroom or in an empty space for five minute can be a huge impact. When you are calmer, you may feel the cravings lessen. You're not in danger if they do since stressful circumstances aren't easy to handle. Just a few minutes can be an important difference in resolving your feelings by eating food or choosing a different method to deal with the issue through meditation and a few minutes in solitude.

Food is a great way to distract yourself. To acknowledge your emotional attachment to food is to recognize it with a sense of mindfulness rather than making an excuse to justify it. It's easy and common to rationalize eating just to ease the stress of a moment or to ease the stress of a stressful situation. There are some emotions that may be traced back in childhood an important event that triggers a reaction to food. In these situations it might take longer to go deeper into our minds to discover the cause of the reaction. Mindfulness assists us in taking the time to look at your body and thoughts at the present moment and pinpointing the root cause of the emotion. Are we experiencing a faster heartbeat, shallow breathing, or something that is causing stomach pain? If someone irritates or offends you, food may soothe the pain temporarily, however, it will manifest in the future when you realize the source of conflict and emotion was not addressed in a way, but instead, resisted by eating.

Some of the pitfalls in Traditional Dieting And How to Avoid It?

Diets don't consider hunger to be an answer, but rather the issue is to avoid your body and adhere to the food plans and restrictions. While many diets today provide a variety of choices, they're identical in that they block the body's natural signals as well as responses to food and hunger. The diets are also able to are based on a reward system of success, which does not relate to your emotions or body, but to the number of inches or pounds you lose. Social media sites often ask users to post photos of themselves before and after that are meant to encourage others to see outcomes and adhere to the diet. But, the opposite outcome or reaction is that people may view as unattainable goals or ones which requires a great deal of effort to attain. The weight loss process is only one part of the struggle, because many people who stick to the diet, even the ones that succeed, get almost all or all of the pounds they lost back. Maintaining the weight loss is a matter of continuing the diet over and over or the risk of gaining weight over time. Exercise can also be a way to sustain the results of a program and is usually considered a necessity instead of a pleasure exercise in itself. It creates a cycle success and failure as people who are dieting fall off the food regimen and or overdo their exercise to make up for it or get back, then have to start the process over from scratch or stop.

Have you tried a variety of diets? How many are you currently trying? If you've tried one diet, it is likely that you've tried a few. The first diet is nearly not successful in the long run , and after this has been completed then you can either stop or try a different one. It's a common pattern people follow with the aim of weight loss for life as well as maintaining healthy living. The focus is on the foods that we consume, and limiting them , without paying attention to the body's signals to us, and not paying attention to our mood and levels of hunger is the most common reason why diets fail. The practice of intuitive eating creates an ongoing pattern of natural eating habits that are in accordance with our thoughts and our body's signals. By being aware of our feelings and reactions to the moment, each whenever we are craving food it will allow us to stop our impulsive response to eat food when we're not hungry and and establish a healthy eating habit that will last for the rest of our lives.

Beware of drastic changes to the Food You Consume

It is possible to learn about the latest diet, cleanse fast or similar to the get-thin-fast fad and testimonies of the success it has. This is a common occurrence for all juice and diet plans however, they can evolve in time. Stay clear of them and focus on what you need. If you're tempted by the idea of go on a diet, remember that it's a reaction to emotion to get a quick result. The most well-known motive for dieting is weight reduction, and there's no specific method that is suitable for every person. However, even with the best results however, there's an limit to the length of time it takes to achieve the desired result. The ability to assess the needs of your body, or evaluate your hunger levels is a problem with diets that aren't compatible with your specific needs, and because of this, it's ideal to avoid them entirely.

Diets create stress and force us to follow an uncompromising plan, which creates the pressure to see results in very short periods of time. It's a way of life that has been around through generations and every new diet promises more results than the previous. The approach to dieting is to put you in the middle of a selection and limit what you are able to pick, regardless of portions carbs, calories or the amount we are permitted to consume food. When we achieve certain milestones and feel determined to stick with the plan or even take a break or "treat" ourselves by having an "cheat" food or similarly restricted foods. This could lead to an increase in pressure to re-enter the diet with more attention and discipline. We disregard the signals that our body is sending us, like cravings for food when it's time to consume food, and we feel guilty for not seeing immediate results.

Chapter 6: Weight Of Not Acceptance

Avoiding emotion through food could be a deliberate tactic or a pattern of eating that's almost inconstant. Also it is possible that you feel an emotion, want to manage it, then whether you are conscious or not using food, you may use it to distract yourself from or modify it, thereby confirming the idea that you cannot handle your emotions.

The process of avoiding or trying to ignore, suppress or alter negative experiences such as thoughts, feelings and bodily sensations causes both emotional distress (Hayes and colleagues. 1996) and emotional eating.

The experience of pain is part of life. We all face emotional pain as well as painful memories and challenges. A lot of people describe their struggle with their emotions as more intense than the physical discomfort. The feeling of discontent with one's body shape and size could be the combination of emotional and physical discomfort. How do you deal with uneasy thoughts feelings, sensations, and feelings?

Control strategies and avoidance are a great way to gain advantages. Our ancestors lived mostly through taking precautions and having some control over their surroundings. These strategies for coping are part of our genes and are not, by themselves, either good or bad. However, they can be sometimes not effective in our daily life. What are the instances when efforts to manage our circumstances successful? If we must focus on a crucial task it's best when we eliminate distractions. If we're looking to lose weight, it's beneficial to limit the consumption of processed and sweet food items at home. However, attempts to manage situations are often unsuccessful in the majority of cases when the rules are too rigid or when we attempt to utilize them in circumstances where they won't work. For instance, if opt to follow a very strict diet that requires you to significantly reduce your consumption of food, you're likely to indulge in the future as you'll be feeling depleted. It is also difficult to control when trying to drastically alter irreversible aspects of the body, for instance, the process of aging. The following exercise is designed to provide you with some experience

69

understanding when strategies for controlling your body could work and the times when they may not be.

Exercise Control or Letting Go?

Spend some time writing about the three instances of situations in which your attempts at controlling the situation do not seem to be working.

Each time you look at a situation take a moment to think of the elements you control and those you aren't able to control.

For instance:

I'm not able to control my feelings of cravings for food.

I don't have control over what people's opinions about me.

I'm not able to control completely how much I love various activities.

I am able to ensure that I buy only the best foods for my home however I am not able to determine what guests or family members decide to bring home.

Certain methods we use for trying to "fix" our emotions can eventually result in us feeling more strongly. Even the most avowed "control freak" is often unsuccessful when it comes to controlling his emotions. You may be able to organize your closets and control your kids but it's quite difficult to shut down your own personal life. Yet, we all are trying to overcome our feelings. Who would want to be overweight, anxious, sad or lonely? However, our best efforts to alleviate emotional pain usually result in an additional burden.

Exercise Let Off Strategies to Avoid

Think about strategies you've used to control your emotions. Have you ever tried to avoid the feeling of being lonely by putting on the television constantly snacking or utilizing other strategies to avoid? Make a list of as many strategies you can, that you've employed to prevent or alter your mood.

What are the feelings that you struggle with the most?

What can you do to practice accepting these emotions?

71

Imagine that you're wearing your favourite pair of suede shoes and you're strolling through the city in search of some important event. It suddenly begins to pour. The awning is up for a while and then you realize that you are wishing away the rain or laying in the shade will not affect the conditions. It is a time to wait, worry, and you become physically tense. Your shoes are going to be destroyed! However, if you delay and don't make it to your appointment your missed opportunity could amount to the cost of a few shoe pairs.

The struggle to control your emotions is similar to making sure your footwear is dry during the rain. It is possible to try, and certain strategies could be effective for a short time--if you're stuck in a rainstorm and you need to get out of the way, it might be beneficial to go inside for a bit of time. But what if you decide to go for a walk or dance in the rain? What if the rain was a part of your daily routine or an anecdote from the meeting, or something (among the numerous things that life gives you) that didn't hinder you?

We aren't able to control our emotions like we regulate the weather. Let's see if we can make ourselves absolutely content today. Tough, isn't it? You can try harder! What do you observe? The emotions of sadness, joy, confusion loss, or confusion--all of them can be turned off or off by us. Willpower is not really effective in this situation. Indeed, any effort to change your mood to the "all happiness every day" channel can often turn your sorrow into genuine misery. What are you trying to accomplish? Why "fail" in a task which isn't likely to happen?

Mark's Story

Mark has been diagnosed as having attention deficit disorder (ADD) as a young child. Naturally, he struggles with his organization and focus. Mark is a sales professional, and due to his ADD He has devised a plan to prepare for meetings, and is systematically analyzing any obstacles that could arise.

One day , while driving to a high-stakes conference, Mark began to sweat. He tried to convince his body to not sweat by imagining the humiliation it would cause to appear to be dripping before his coworkers. This only led to further sweating. Even more disturbing, Mark felt so uncomfortable and stressed that he purchased a large cold beer and a cheeseburger despite the fact that Mark was headed to a business event and had high cholesterol.

Mark's efforts to manage anxiety and manage his body was not working at times, and it wasn't for his first experience. He had a well-thought out plan to deal with meetings, yet he feeling exhausted both before and after meetings. He tried to calm himself by eating comfort food as well as television and alcohol. You can imagine that the more time he spent in regulating his body and avoiding anxious thoughts, the more stressed was he really felt and the less effective at his job. In the event of the day I've mentioned the more he sweated emotionally as well as physically. This is a powerful metaphor for the futility of our efforts to control the uncontrollable could be.

The hid feelings cause you to Feel more

Although you might limit the way you express emotion, you will experience more sensations as a result of attempts to control the emotions (Gross and Levenson, 1997). If, for instance, you attempt to keep from feeling anxious, you could decrease the expression of anxiety that you display on your face a certain extent however your heart rate will rise due to your trying to appear calm. Therefore, limiting the emotional expression will offer relief from the feelings and can actually cause the opposite. Researchers (e.g., Wegner, Quillian Houston, and Houston 1996) are also concerned that attempting to block emotions can hinder your ability to manage information. Imagine this that if you're focusing on controlling your emotions it's hard to focus on and pay attention to the world around you. In the case of Mark it is possible that he's too focused on his efforts to appear calm that he is unable to observe how engaged his coworkers are in his presentation. Repressing your emotions can affect your relationships with other people. If you control your behavior, will the people who are around you be aware of the struggle? With your focus in controlling how you present yourself are you likely to have a lot of a chance to see the things that are happening with them? Most likely not and the effect is that you'll likely feel more and more isolated , and less likely to display loving and supportive behavior.

Feel Less, Eat More?

How can suppressing emotion cause a rise in consumption of comfort food items? It is possible that the act of suppressing can deplete your emotional reserves. It is possible that you are focusing in repressing your emotions which leaves you with very few options for being aware of your diet (Vohs as well as Heatherton 2000). In fact, if you're not following a diet plan it is much less inclined to indulge because there is less pressure on your the choices you make regarding food.

Here's the pattern When you start feeling sad, it's normal. It is difficult to express your feelings however, you try to let it go. You're now less in control in eating what you want to eat, and tend to eat unhealthy comfort food items. And then, you are feeling guilty when you choose to choose to eat comfort food, which is a negative feeling! What happens when you are unable to suppress the guilt? If you have rigid expectations of perfection, or refuse to accept yourself for who your true self, food can serve as a means of escape (Heatherton and Baumeister 1991) However, escaping only once can make it more likely to look for escape again and again, and forgetting that this method doesn't last long.

What could occur if you did not have to escape by eating? What could happen if gently acknowledged and confronted your grief?

Chapter 7: The Most Important Things You Need

To Know About Your Emotional Brain

It is a mighty Rapid-Response System that is Highly Effective and Rapid-Response

The brain that is emotional the first to be next in line, after the brainstem to take in the most the sensory information that comes in. Because it's equipped to deal with life-threatening situations in a hostile situation, its response speed is higher than the cortex.

Since it is more crucial for immediate survival It has the ability to completely override the cortex in the event that it is activated sufficiently. If you are in a situation where stopping to think might be the reason you killed it is a great option. One of the practical aspects is that the brain's emotional part will begin to respond to information that is coming in and shut in the cortex prior to it is even able to play.

When you are confronted with a tempting food items isn't a life-or-death occasion, but it could trigger intense reactivity in the brain's emotional system in the same. Any event that triggers the emotions brain -- whether it's smell, sight or mention or thinking about certain foods--can trigger the mechanisms that eventually block the cortex.

In order to be successful with food management in the current world it is essential to minimize conditions where your brain's emotional part starts to spin and overtake your cortex is able to take over the situation.

The present is prioritized.

The wild life is about living the present moment and assisting one's children succeed, and so the brain's emotional system is fixed to the moment. It doesn't readily make sense of delayed effects, and is not averse to delayed gratification. These inputs are far too distant from the present to stimulate it in a meaningful way.

It is most responsive to the most immediate stimulus that's why it is so enthralled by the trigger food, instead of to the more abstract results in the future. The debate that is going on inside your head could read as, This will be amazing! I can't wait! Vs. I'm always in a state of self-doubt when I eat this way. Isn't that enough to cause me to stop wanting to take it on? ?

It is important to note that although the emotional brain isn't affected by future outcomes but it's your emotional mind that will be experiencing them once the time is right. This is where you feel the pain that is caused by narrow-sighted and impulsive decisions.

It's the place where you celebrate happiness and satisfaction when things turn out to be a success.

Due to the limitations mentioned above, however the emotional brain isn't able to prioritise future results when making choices; in the same way, it doesn't discern where it's headed. Only the cortex can perceive the future, and only the cortex is able to determine what options can make the brain feel the most happy present and in the near future.

It develops strong Biases

If you've found something you like, that particular experience or item is put into that "like it and want to repeat it" category, possibly very strongly. You'll give the experience benefit of doubt going forward, identifying it as a positive thing since you liked it previously.

Since it's nice to be able to work out a solution and not need to think about it all over again It's a good idea to stay with this mentality. Therefore, you'll be inclined to minimize, rationalize, denial or even ignore evidence that is contrary to your initial assessment.

Think about what happens after you've found a favourite food such as. Let's say the food is something that makes you satisfied just by contemplating this, then you eat it in every way you could. You discover that your favorite food contains some ingredients that are a bit scary. It's natural to walk away however this isn't the case. You are a fan of the food, so you comfort yourself by rationalizing, "They wouldn't sell it even if it were harmful to the human body," or "I eat lots of other foods that are healthier , so everything is balanced," or "This is commonplace, everybody eats this."

If you've heard about the same ingredients that are questionable in a dish that you've not previously tried, you could be able to pass the item off. Because it's a dish you're already familiar with but the mind-sets begin. The food is a part of your diet and then try to be a bit more careful and not think of it. The emotions can overpower facts.1

What happens when you start to realize that when you eat certain foods that are loved by everyone typically, you're feeling miserable, stuffed and feeling miserable? It's logical to leave any food that is likely to make you feel unsatisfied and disgusting. Who would want to? In this instance it's unlikely. Your mind's emotional part has been fixated on these food items as something it is aspires to and is based on how pleasant you think you will have while your eating them. It will be difficult to provide enough evidence to prompt your mind to rethink this stance, as emotions are a lot more powerful than facts.

The emotional brain's ability to develop stubborn biases can show through in a variety of ways, above or beyond food issues.2 Addiction, for instance it has to do with part with the emotion brain classifying something as highly appealing, and then relentlessly seeking it, even when there is no anticipated reward. That is, you're performing a task that isn't providing the reward you expected and yet you're strongly compelled to continue since it seems as if that reward is likely to come when you try for it long enough.

The emotional brain can cling to an old belief system such as this even in the face of numerous different experiences, but they do not support it. It is common to continue believing instead of destroying the mental structure that is in place and creating something completely new. This is the reason we continue to rely on food in spite of ourselves.

Phobias On the other hand tend to be a result of the brain's emotional response to an event as a threat and then avoid it, even in the absence of any harm. The brain's emotional part will hold on to fear despite the fact that things are always turning out fine and feelings prevail and again.

Aversions are smaller than phobias but they are a good instance of the brain's emotional classifying something as negative despite evidence that suggests that it is not.

There are many people who feel resentful to the concept of healthy diet and exercise routines, for example, despite the fact that both produce positive outcomes. In this instance the mind of the emotional believes that these activities are heavy rather than rewarding due to the fact that the rewards do not arrive in a timely manner and, even more so due to the effort needed upfront. The emotional brain is able to maintain this view despite the fact contrary to this, and with only a few minutes they can bring more joy and satisfaction than other options.

It's got a long Memory

The brain's emotional component tends to prefer the familiar--"the one you know"--to the unfamiliar even if it isn't without its drawbacks. This is the reason you might resist trying healthier habits even when you realize you require them. You resist them because they're different. This is why you could abandon the patterns at some point in the future even though they've been working well for you. Some part of you would like to return to familiar patterns even though it was the cause of the problems that prompted you to changing in the first place. A brief look at the functioning of the nervous system will help you understand why we experience these tendencies.

When you think, or do something, it's accomplished through sending electrical signals through the nervous system. The signals travel between the one neuron (neuron) one to another, triggering the bodily systems that are required to carry out the action you've chosen to undertake.

Similar to a path in the woods that gets more easily to locate with each usage, neural pathways get stronger through practice.3 The more solid your neural pathways, the easier and effectively you can complete this particular task. That's why you need to practice to become perfect, but also the reason that the old habits are hard to break.

Overeating habits have been tested hundreds of times over the course of many years, resulting in neural superhighways that allow for their function.

When you begin to build new neural pathways to create better outcomes the old ones go into obscurity, but they do not disappear. The older pathways are still in place, well-constructed but not active, right alongside the more modern ones that are more effective however they are in the process of being built.

In daily life, this implies that if you stop opting for the latest path it will automatically return to the path you've mastered.

It can be done effortlessly that you're not aware of it. You might be "finding" yourself in the middle of eating a portion of cookies, heading to a drive-through or completing the kids' leftovers. The transition to the previous pattern isn't as smooth and happens within a matter of seconds.

It is possible to imagine the day you completely forget the past difficult days of addiction, but the fact lies in the fact that your neural pathway that lead to it will never go out of place. This is the reason why the chance of relapse is usually an extent for the duration of a lifetime. Be extremely cautious when you start thinking that you should be able to accomplish this now in a safe manner.

However, this doesn't mean that all you need to be looking forward to is going through the rest time, just one white-knuckled, day at a. These new neural pathways in the event that you've put them in the right spots can allow you to relax and live your life to the fullest then ever.

Also, it isn't an absolute requirement that you perform flawlessly is required to be successful. In the moment, lapses in performance are to be anticipated, however they must be treated with a sense of urgency. A mistake--any action that you didn't anticipate you could not control, or that ultimately left you any point unhappy that if you'ren't more prudent in the future it's likely that things will become worse.

A food complication is similar to driving in a car and veering from your path until you come to bump strips that run along the edges. There's nothing really bad that happens however, you've been warned that something is happening more quickly than normal. Don't ignore the warnings to your risk.

There's a chance that you'll have lapses -- hopefully smaller ones, for the duration in your existence. Take note of the warning signs you can learn how much you possibly can about them. When properly studied, each will make you stronger. As time passes, you'll encounter these issues less often and recover faster, but the odds are they'll pop occasionally. The best solution is to continue to learn and progressing.

It's not very well matched to the World of today.

There is a vast difference between what helps us survive when in nature and the things that improves it in the modern world. This means that our well-being is at risk with the same behaviors which have protected us for the majority of our time.

Our love of sweets is an excellent example of how it is a great choice in nature, exposing us to the essential nutrients. Today this similar taste preference can lead us to indulgence in sweets which can trigger a variety of diseases as well as addictive behaviors.

The issue is how to harness the energy of the brain's emotional part so that it can again produce positive outcomes instead of harmful ones despite living in a non-natural environment that continuously bombards it with inaccurate information.

It's a lot easier to take on if you are able to keep track of what your brain is doing for you, regardless of its peculiar quirks and flaws.

It's Still Why Life is worth living

Have you ever felt a connection with someone, or experienced the warm feeling of knowing that that someone is in love with you? Have you got a passion or passion that you are looking forward to and that captivates you so you can't keep your mind while doing it? Have you ever experienced the excitement of an unanticipated amazing delight? Do you feel a surge of confidence after overcoming the challenge you didn't think you were capable of tackling? Did you have an experience that was flawless?

These events and many others similar experiences come through your emotional brain as it is the place the area where your emotions develop. It's not just an area of happiness and happiness, though it's also a place where all the suffering in your life is also felt there as does guilt, shame, and guilt of eating too much.

Many people, when they learn that a certain part of the brain is responsible for the habit of eating, have an overwhelming desire to have the part removed surgically. If it were to happen it would mean you'd never experience any of the emotions that create a multi-dimensional existence. Imagine a world where everything is a blur. Would you really wish for that?

The goal, then, is to recognize the things your brain's emotional intelligence makes possible, while also learning how to utilize it and take control of it better in accordance with the strange demands of the present. If you're able to do that you'll see that your emotional brain can become the source of greater happiness, peace and genuine happiness than it has ever been before.

Unexpected dangers of Modern Life

The modern world offers a wealth of opportunities and poses an enormous mental challenge for the brain's emotional. Once you are aware of how it operates and how it works, you can arrange for your lifestyle to become more calming, simpler, fulfilling, and even more pleasurable.

Problem of Too Much Problem of Too Much

The emotional brain is designed towards rapid judgment of things in the world and swift decision-making based on this judgement. In the face of limited options and resources it is evident that the "get whatever you can when you are able to" system is effective. There is no requirement for self-regulation of behavior in the world of nature because there's not much possibility of acquiring more of any type.

It's not that we're not capable of self-regulation. The issue is that the capacity for self-regulation is not in the brain of our emotions which has the greatest power of immediate in the way that decisions are taken.

We are constantly able to access delicious food. The brain's emotional response to this abundance the same way it does to the limited opportunities to which it has adjusted: striving to have everything. It's not normal to be able to eat food and the physical capacity to eat more and yet decide to cut down on eating. The brain that is emotional does not work this way.

Food isn't the only subject in the field where this issue is played out. With the tendency of the emotional brain for instant gratification and taking advantage of opportunities that are immediate generally it's easy to recognize how abundant and easy opportunities of every kind can go off track.

Take a look at other activities that are associated with a possibility of becoming addicted including alcohol and sexual activity, smoking on gambling, online activities. It is certainly possible to engage in one of these without falling into self-destructive behavior, and many do, however, a large majority fail in trying. In such situations shows that you've got an emotional brain that is unintentionally self-destructing when it applies the "get everything you can" strategy to situations that allows you to overdo it. "Enough" does not belong to an emotion brain concept. The emotional brain when in its own way cannot cease until negative effects of excess are difficult to continue, or until there is no other option.

The mighty, defenseless emotional Brain

The cortex has the ability to easily offer the self-regulation that makes it feasible for brain's emotional part to live happily and healthy in the midst of many.

The issue is that the brain's emotional part is constantly activated by opportunities and triggers to create uncontrollable power grab, which locks in the cortex. In the event of this happening then the brain's emotional system is in a state of confusion and cannot defend itself. Anger, chaos as well as regret, are the expected outcome.

The need for constant self-management that is deliberate and systematic is not new to humanity as a whole however its importance increases every year. The need for it today is far greater than what it was 40 to fifty years ago or throughout the history of humanity before the present. It's perhaps not surprising that it's been difficult for a lot individuals to comprehend the changes is needed to be a successful person in the very different environment of today.

At the time of writing, reality television is a well-established field with a subset dedicated for survival, with limited support. The shows demonstrate how useful our drives remain after we've returned to an environment that is suitable for them. Cast members are exactly like we'd like to be doing: eat whatever they can get their hands on and sleep whenever they want to. The location they are in provides little chances to eat and rest, thus promoting the survival of the fittest.

In our world, where there is endless opportunities for both, same choices endanger thousands of people's lives.

Self-Management for the Life

It is crucial to grasp the chasm between the way our brains function and the needs of the environment in which we live. Our survival instincts when left unchecked in a world of excess, can lead to behaviors that encourage self-destruct instead of survival.

We're well-equipped to manage this issue in the event that we keep the cortex occupied. What can we do to achieve this? The answer lies in enhancing the cortex so that it becomes better in controlling the emotional brain, since that's just not feasible.

What is effective is keeping the brain's emotional state calm enough to be open to more advanced strategies. It's when the emotional brain is reactive, as in anticipation, excitement and anxiety, depression or anger, that it may begin to take over the cortex. This is the reason the logic of the brain isn't enough to get rid of an overwhelming craving to consume food.

If you are living in a world of simple food, it is essential to be aware and deliberate about the food you eat within your daily life. It's not an act of punishment or burden, it is simply a necessary aspect of the way we live. Your brain's emotional part will always be on alert ready to leap into action by using the old drives if you trigger it too frequently. The only way to prevent this is to reduce the amount that occurs.

Beating the Diet Mentality

This book promotes a non-diet approach for weight loss that is in the against our conditioned. Dieting is a staple in our society to the point that it is mandatory. Do you remember the days that you ate whenever you felt hungry, and didn't think about weight, calories or health, or even the way you looked? If you're anything like me, it was a long time ago. It's not even our responsibility. Many forces are working to make us feel unhappy and discontented with the way we look and how we consume food. One of the main causes is the multitude of diets that are competing for attention, and money.

Review your dieting history. What are the number of diets you've been on? Are you currently on one? The study I conducted found that people were currently eating the diet for about 38 percent of their lives. Many beginning their diets as early as 5 years old! The negative effects of this early exposure to diets ranges from feeling overweight to being unhappy about the way we look.

Diets aren't working

It's easy to be attracted by promises of astonishing results in just 30 days, the diet your friend is currently testing, or the claim that you'll become smarter more powerful, healthier, and happier by using a certain product. It is obvious that the outcomes you want will require some patience and work, however, you are still tempted to look for a quick solution. Your only hope is that you'll get your ideal shape or better health and fitness, and it will be done quickly and easily. However, let's be real with one another. If one of the diets you've tried on were productive (however you define it) Would you be taking this book?

Diets in particular haven't done much to aid in weight loss or curb appetite. According to research suggests. The rates of obesity in America are among the most high anywhere in the world. Many people are on diets, however, nearly two-thirds of US adults are obese or overweight and these figures and the size of their waists are increasing (Ogden and co. 2014). There's a multibillion-dollar world weight loss industry based on the notion that you'll require its diet supplements for a long period of time.

Researchers from The University of California, Los Angeles studied the results of thirty-one long-term studies on diets. They concluded that, although dieters may lose weight at first most people on diets gain the weight back, and more. "Yo-yo" people who shed and gain weight repeatedly can increase the risk for hypertension, diabetes heart metabolic syndrome, and other diseases (Mann and colleagues. 2007). This study of the literature shows that you're actually better off not going to a diet in beginning.

There are numerous anecdotal stories of poor diet failures. Stacey is a dieter who has been around for a long time has stated that "I have been on a number of diets since I was 15 years old. I am able to determine the amount of calories in any foods." She confirmed the findings of research: "Diets never worked out. Whatever diet I've ever tried, it was never ever permanent. I would constantly weigh myself and my weight always returned."

As Stacey Many dieters are unhappy and have thrown their hands in displeasure. Paula has said, "Because of my diet experiences, I've reached a stage where I don't even feel capable of doing it. The most adolescent advice about the world can't inspire me at this moment. I've tried nearly every diet imaginable and that isn't a method I would like to live my life. I am among those who when they hear the word "diet" and then eat every food item you can think of."

If you're an individual who doesn't adhere to a strict diet, you could be shocked at how affected by the diet-related mindset. You claim that you don't follow an eating plan however, you secretly fear those times that your food choices aren't yours to control. You examine the food you consume before eating it, you categorize food items in terms of "good" or "bad," or you have lots of musts and don'ts when it comes to food. It's possible that you would like to be healthier but you're not allowing you enjoyment of food when it isn't in"the "good" class. (Note that there is some difference between a diet-based mentality and being conscious of deciding whether you desire to eat certain food items after a thorough examination of their flavor and impact to your physique.) Due to their ubiquitous nature diet-related ideas and images are instilled into us all.

Make a point now to check in with yourself. Although this book is an essentially "non-diet" method You may be thinking that it's the next diet that actually succeed. Be truthful about yourself. "Dieting mind "dieting mentality" is very smart.

Why Diets Aren't Working

Why don't diets perform? The first reason is that diets severely restrict what foods you can eat or the amount of food you can consume and you won't be able to eating this way in the long run. Consuming a small amount of foods or eating low calories can aid in losing weight while on the diet, but once you stop following it and eat as you usually do (which you'll) then you'll gain the weight back.

Thirdly, what happens when you say you'll never get a meal? You'd love it! Right? If you do finally manage to get it, you'll be eating plenty. Sometimes, you'll eat the food you're forbidden to eat in private, while nobody is watching. You'll consume it at a rapid pace so that nobody can see your face. You'll need to consume lots of it since you think you're not going to get it ever again.

My friend Lynn would not let herself indulge in sweets and candy at home and would then steal these treats from the drawers on her desks of colleagues. It was not a very smart idea since all her colleagues knew she did it. They happily stocked their cupboards to let her steal pleasure. Janice who was twenty-five years old, an athlete who would only sneak in sweets and cookies during work hours because her husband, who was a professional athlete, was trying to keep her in a strict diet of carbs and calories. Both women could not be denied, however they did not really indulge in their desserts, as they were with their friends and family in the privacy of their homes.

Fourth, when you're depending only on an external source (such as diet plans) to inform you of what you should eat, it's not listening the wisdom and knowledge of your body. When you're not able to begin listening to your own inner wisdom (instead of an eating plan) regarding what, when, when and why and how much consume, it's unlikely that you'll be able to alter your diet. The body has incredible sensors for what foods are healthy, which foods are harmful to your body and the amount of food you should consume, and what nutrients it requires. Wild animals consume and live their lives according to instinctual internal guidance and search the forest and fields to find food sources that fulfill their nutritional needs. There was no need to teach them a nutrition education but they are incredibly adept at being aware of what they should consume. Humans are more nimble than animals, however the majority of people have separated themselves from the body's natural instincts.

This leads me to my final and possibly most important aspect that diets can eliminate the joy of food. If you are on a diet, your sole joy is when you do something wrong, and you will! My belief has always been that food should be an amazing element of our lives that should be enjoyed, and enjoyed. A diet-free approach to weight loss is one that recognizes the joy of eating food of all kinds. If you really enjoy your food, it is slowing down to enjoy the moment and relish the sweetness of life.

Starting steps to take

In your mouth, under your stomach and on your tongue in your eyes, within your brain, you have the necessary knowledge to be educated on the best time, place and how much you should consume. Instead of eating food to cure or hide your feelings You will be able to face difficult times with compassion and aplomb. It will help you identify the mindsets and beliefs that hinder your efforts to eat healthier and healthier, so that you can be in the driving seat in making decisions on what you eat and how you live your life. Alongside the change in the way you think about food, you'll also gain an appreciation towards your own body (no regardless of how big you are) that will encourage you to be more mindful of it.

Before you get any further Here are a few points I'd like you take into consideration that will assist you in turning your attention on yourself.

1. Stop the Diets

If you're not currently in a diet, good. By not attempting to lose weight, you have the chance to identify your own internal sources of wisdom.

If your physician is recommending a particular diet for medical reasons be sure to stay with it. The knowledge you acquire will allow you to feel more confident about, achieve your diet, and be happy with the one you're on.

2. Take a step back from the Scale

Whatever anxiety it may create for you I'd like you to allow yourself to see what staying away from the scale will teach you about. Don't rely on an external scale to measure your weight will help you start your journey to the inside. It is the initial step towards paying attention to your internal signals to determine the way you eat. Additionally, you can tell if you're the difference between being heavier or lighter by looking at the way your body appears and feels , or whether or not the pants you wear.

Do you think that getting on the scale been a helpful way to lose weight? Are you always satisfied with the numbers that you see on your scale? I've asked this question to numerous people and the majority of them say an emphatic no. Being off the scale means you not create one moment in each day that you intentionally find yourself feeling disappointed.

Personally, my strategy with the weight scales was establish an amount I wanted but couldn't achieve it. It took a while before an amazing thing happened. Finally, I astonishingly achieved my goals. I was so content for about just two minutes (literally)--before I realized that I had to shed five pounds! Some time ago, I got off the scales with my ex-husband and have been happier than since then.

The main reason for not weighting yourself a challenge is going to the doctor's office, as the first thing you're required to do is step onto the scale. After dealing with this issue for many years, here's my suggestion: inform the nurse that you'll get on the scale, but that you're not interested in knowing the weight you are carrying. If you take a look at it, the majority of the time the weight is in kilograms. If you're not adept in converting kilograms to pounds, you'll never know the weight of your body. I've admitted to being an outspoken rebel in the past, and refused to step on the scale. However, I've been advised by a physician that keeping your weight each time you check-up is required for insurance providers and Medicaid. It's best to be considerate and allow them to weigh you.

3. Make a Goal (Besides the Weight Loss) to start you off.

For the moment, I would like to encourage you to take your focus away from a number on a scale. The number is just an external confirmation of what you're about and how you wish to feel. Therefore, I'd like to urge you to move further away from your goal of losing weight. Also, how do you want to be performing or thinking differently, which could ultimately result in losing weight?

Stop for a few seconds and relax your eyes while you take a few deep breaths. Find out what questions come up. The most frequent responses

I hear include "I'd like to eat more slowly," "I'd like to stop eating when I'm fully satisfied," "I'd like to quit eating at the computer or while doing my reading" as well as "I'd like to quit eating the last bites of food that are on the plates of my children."

If you don't have any thoughts at this point, you can keep checking to see what happens as you read.

Building Realistic confidence

Now! Please, drum roll answer the question that every motivational pep talk I've ever heard of asks what's the difference between people who are successful in achieving an objective, like urge surfing as opposed to the ones who fail? I don't think I know answers to this difficult question. Let's take a moment to consider: What hinders actions? What could be the potential solutions?

Think about it: one of your enduring objectives is to complete the marathon of 26 miles, which is a distance of twenty-six miles. What are the steps you must take to reach the level of physical fitness you'll need before you are able to run the marathon? Based on Olympic professional and coach for runners Jeff Galloway, to prep for the marathon, you start by walking or running for 30 minutes, two times each week. You then carefully build up your endurance as time goes on. In just twenty-nine weeks you'll go from incapable of running more than 3 miles to running 26 miles. This isn't an after-hours informational video; this is an instructional program that thousands of runners like me and you have completed to make marathon running an achievable goal. To build confidence, thenbreak down a project into manageable pieces. To build a sense confidence in general, you should regularly test yourself.

We all face problems. The definition of mastery is performing tasks that allow you to feel confident as well as confident (e.g., Linehan 1993b). Self-efficacy, or the beliefs you hold regarding your abilities, have an enormous influence on your life. You develop your belief in self-efficacy by mastering. Some wait until they are confident enough to take on a challenge. What's alternative? Enhance your competence by carefully selecting goals that are challenging and achievable. You should ask yourself "Where is my goal located on the spectrum of effortless to impossibly difficult?" Mastery is all about being at the middle of that spectrum.

Nearly every successful program that helps you alter the way you conduct yourself is a sensible step that will give you hope to move on to next step. Consider Alcoholics Anonymous, whose motto is "One day at an moment," not "Don't drink for the remainder the rest of your existence." It is likely that this kind of attitude will cause anxiety, which could cause drinking to increase, whereas the former one is to be manageable and improves the likelihood of abstinence. One of my patients described mastery development as "tricking your brain" by avoiding routes that can lead to resistance. I view taking actionable actions as the best method to develop confidence and prepare yourself to change the way you interact between your food and your emotions.

Mastery and Urge surfing

It is essential to have an attitude of mastery and the urge to surf builds mastery. Being aware that you've trained to the point to be able to run a marathon gives you an element of self-confidence in various other aspects. "Of course I've ridden the desire to order nachos, I've experienced many urges to give up exercising!" Similarly, repeatedly searching for the urge to purchase nachos could also build an overall sense of self-confidence and the belief that you'll be able to resist the next temptation to eat.

If your mind is sending to you the signal "Give up! Do you really need to bother?" you can thank your mind for the thought. A way to thank the mind of a thought is watching the thought with no judgment instead of responding to the thought like it's a true alarm. After that, you can encourage yourself up by reliving unpleasant urges that you've have ridden. Similarly, practicing urge surfing builds mastery. By constantly observing how you label, identify, and ride the urges, you'll build self-confidence in the ability of allow yourself more time between desire and actions.

A lot of people with eating issues make eating the primary focus of their life. You might feel that you've done everything you can to avoid eating out of anger. Maybe taking a step back and seeing the ways you excel at other aspects will give you the confidence to believe that you'll be able to end your eating disorder. We don't have the motivation to set goals if we do not believe we'll achieve these goals.

The ability to master different aspects of your life could decrease your vulnerability to extreme emotional and impulsive. For instance, your desire to give the most humorous toast to your friend's wedding creating stress. By taking a class on speech-making with the intention of improving your public speaking abilities and conquering your fear could help you reduce the anxiety you are experiencing. Furthermore, when you think through your problems and work to improve the confidence of your audience, then you might be less inclined to resort towards food to help ease anxiety about your speech. Knowing that you can feel uncomfortable (for instance, ignoring the urge to fake laryngitis so that you don't give the toast) could affect your ability to withstand the desire to take a bite.

A Purposeful Use of Pain

To build muscle mastery, you must do resistance training. We'll be honest. The idea of running to improve your daily mileage is (literally) not a stroll on the beach. The goal isn't instant gratification. game here (nor will it get your long). Learning, as a rule, cannot be achieved in a single moment.

In the short run mastery requires a lot of perseverance. Long-term mastery can boost your mood and decrease the likelihood of being affected by negative emotions. As time passes, engaging in rigorous activities will increase your self-esteem and decrease the feeling of depressed. People typically report the feeling of joy that comes from accomplishment rather than seeking immediate satisfaction. Perhaps you are having a hard time boosting your self-esteem, doubting your capacity to feel a sense satisfaction, or eating in order to calm your nerves. You could alter your mood by doing. If your thoughts try to convince you to not be concerned about ignoring your desires and handling your emotions in a different manner or enhancing your musical skills, be aware of the thoughts, and let them drift in the background like all the other noise. By altering your habits and habits, you'll be free of. The raucous dissonance of your thoughts could slow down. In the end, you complete the marathon on your legs and not with your thoughts. It would be great to have your thoughts assist you on your way however, it's not essential. Are you willing to shift your body to what you value to you and pay focus there?

People may visit an Zen Ashram to improve their spiritual. They can meditate. They also clean floors. Spend money, go to a hill to sit and meditate and clean toilets. In the past I was fortunate enough to take part in an enlightenment retreat with Marsha Linehan who was the psychologist behind DBT situated in Tucson, Arizona. I imagined a relaxing time at the pool, enjoying the vegetarian meals, gaining mindfulness and becoming a more compassionate person in only five days. I had no idea that I would be facing an early time of 5:30 a.m. rise-up to sit for six hours every day in front of an unpainted wall, or cleaning. These tasks all required mental acuity. After a long day of looking at the wall, I broke my habit of silence and I asked Marsha to see if it would be possible to sit in the sun and look at the Cacti. She replied something similar to "Life is all about what happens when you're dealing with walls that are white." Aiming for only enjoyment, or at a minimum easy steps to growth can slow our advancement. So, the challenges that we encounter along the way can be beneficial. A concierge or room service are not going to change your mood the same way as accomplishments can change the way you experience life and your perception of self.

The Motivation Myth

"You are not able to urge surfers or prepare for a marathon until you're driven." This statement is a popular myth. Motivation is similar to winning the lottery. It is not a sure thing and it isn't a guarantee of a fulfilling life. You might think that you are a good person and do your best work when you are motivated. Do you get up to go to work or wash your clothes? Do you feel inspired to complete those tasks regularly? Of course, when we feel a rush of inspiration, the enthusiasm fades away. If you wait to experience a different feeling than you already feel will result in waiting for a long period of time. Consciously acting, repeatedly and repeatedly, will result in mastery.

Let's be clear:

1. Motivation isn't a condition to take action.

2. Action is the catalyst for actions.

3. Motivation would be great.

Exercise: Building mastery step by step

1. Set a goal to complete at least one thing every day to feel an appreciation of your accomplishment. You could meditate or a dance class, or read the classic you've been reading but have stopped after college, or even urge yourself to surf.

2. When you are engaged in mastery muscle building, pay attention. Be aware of what you are doing and be focused on it. Three miles is just (and completely) mile three. It's not counting down to mile 26. There is no need to analyse your

performance. Don't be a judge. This is the perfect opportunity to expand your perspective of what you believe to be feasible. Cheer yourself on.

3. Increase the complexity of the goal you want to achieve as time passes.

Practicing Nonjudgmental Mastery

The concept of nonjudgmental mastery could be an untruth. How can you be aware of growing and becoming more proficient if you don't have a judgment? In the same way, not having judgmental desires may be counterintuitive. The truth is the exact opposite of judgment. "I have run five miles in the last week, and last week I ran 4 miles" isn't a judgement but a matter of fact. In the same way, observing, "I sat with my emotions" can also be a declaration of fact. It is not about an act of judging and can be free from the psychological consequences of being judged. If you think of yourself as having experienced an "bad" run what are the chances to go back to the track, or to notice the improvement in your mood? In the same way, labeling your urges as "bad" can intensify your struggles. However, taking a look at, "Is engaging in this desire beneficial?" may facilitate positive actions.

The goal of mastery isn't to remove an emotional state that is negative or to avoid a new one. In attempting to force yourself experience something different from what you currently feel will keep feeling X, and create feelings Y. You are feeling sad, and you begin working on an New York Times crossword puzzle and you wish you felt better. Then you're feeling sad and angry. It is possible to notice that the sadness in your body and accepting that feeling and fully participating in the crossword game in the interest of mastery but not to hide the sadness.

Chapter 8: Sustainability Strategies To Practice

Intuitive Eating

When you see how efficient the intuitive way of eating can be in keeping your weight in check and maintaining general good health, chances that you'll want to start it immediately. Although that's what we want, it's crucial to remember that no path is without challenges. You may, for instance, be surrounded by people asking you to join their weight loss plan. While you may not wish to appear cocky however, you have to make sure you are firm on the path to better health you'd like to embark on. It is important to be able to inform your friends and colleagues that you are aware of the necessity to shed weight, but have found a more efficient method and a less stressful method. They might actually want to be a part of your team instead.

However, you can confront your own personal struggles which you'll need to find a method of taking on.

Below are some suggestions to make sure you stay unwavering on the path of eating intuitively:

1.Practice Hara hachi bu

What, in the interest of eating healthily does that mean? Actually, it's a phrase from the Okinawans of Japan which relates to the best way to determine the time you should stop eating. What is the Okinawans typically mean by this phrase is the have to stop eating once you're 80percent full. This is the 20-minute gap between the stomach and your mouth which the Okinawa principle appears to connect to.

It is believed that this attitude of the Okinawas is having an impact on their health, since they are believed to be the most healthy group of humans on the planet. The age of 100 is not a big issue for someone from Okinawa. In reality, the average man living on the island lives to be 78 years old, while the average female lives all the way to 86 years. The main point is to take your time eating enough but and not too much. Be satisfied, but not overstuffed.

2.Do do not classify food good or bad.

Isn't the saying says too much of something could be harmful? The wise say that the Bible is a good source as well as professionals have backed it up. Be careful not to find specific foods , as they're the ones you think are acceptable, and displaying such a an attitude of resentment towards certain foods because you think they are bad that you're prone to developing goose pimples when you come across them. It can be extremely stressful. What happens when stress is present? The cortisol hormone and its weight-gain catalyzing function begins to take over, anxiety grows and you become distracted from the primary task of being aware of your body.

It is important to note that no one advocates recklessness. In fact, it's well-known that fibrous foods and whole meals are beneficial for the body, and they cannot alter the biology of our bodies. They assist in keeping blood sugar levels at healthy levels and keep the liver functioning optimally. Therefore, it is a good idea to take these.

The most successful way to eat intuitively is get rid of being too concerned about the food they put into their bodies. Dietary stricters take time to identify different sources of fibre, usually labeling arrow roots as sweet potatoes as unhealthy since they're carbohydrates. For those who are intuitive"This is food that is not processed and my body is craving it, so let it go. In this way, you'll feel free and your taste buds will feel well and your body won't feel a need to eat. So, your stomach and the taste buds reach an equilibrium and the result will be a content and healthy you.

3.Identify your interests and then practice them

A mind that is idle, as someone told me is the place where the devil works. In our situation the devil is the need to eat just to pass the time. Actually, it's when you're sitting and not resting, but actually unoccupied - that you start to think about all the things that aren't working out for you. It's as if everyone's life is flawless! Once the negatives start flow, the only thing that can help is food. Be aware that no matter how healthy the food item however, the body will not need it while you consume it, you'll be harming your health.

That's why you have to find something you can do to prevent you from emotionally eating. What about going for a walk and enjoying the beauty of nature? It's not just healthy to breathe clean air but also a moderate amount of exercising is always appreciated. In the end, eating intuitively isn't a reason to stop engaging in other healthy activities like engaging in exercise or keeping company of positive people.

4. Be honest about your distractions

Anyone who said anything about serving two masters was correct. There is a chance that you will cause a rift with one. In our instance the ideal setting for eating intuitively is one in which the TV is turned off and you don't have your laptop open prior to you eat. Also, reading your messages on your phone while you eat is not a good idea.

Did we talk about becoming more attuned with your body? It is only possible to do this by focusing your attention at the body. It willthen be very simple for you to recognize the signals of satiety and to stop exactly where the Okinawas would. When your brain has completed registering the entire amount of food that's entered your stomach, your brain won't let your stomach know that it is full; instead, it will give

122

you a nod and tell you that you're no longer hungry.

In the end front, it's the freedom that comes from eating intuitively that makes you a hero. You'll know you're on the right path when you don't shiver when someone offers you food items that aren't yours at a party or not scold your friends for having unhealthy snacks in their presence. You will have control and you won't be tempted to indulge in the event that your body is not craving the food. You'll be fueled by the condition of your body and your mind and not what your eyes see.

Chapter 9: Strategies For Hands-On Use To

Prevent And Overcome Binge Eating

If you are struggling with eating disorders, you are aware of how easy it is that you turn your attention to food when there's a problem with your life. Instead of gaining weight and calories Here are some practical ways to stop the cycle of binge eating.

Managing Stress

Stress is among the main triggers for people who eat a lot. When life gets difficult and it's tempting to head to the fridge or go for a drive through the drive-through in order to order a large portion from fast-food. Instead of making food your solution next time you feel like life's challenges weigh you down look for other avenues to relieve your anxiety. Exercise is among the most effective options, engaging you and helping you remain in good shape. You can set up a regular program that eases tension on a regular basis. Think about visiting the massage therapist or picking yoga classes to break the hold of tension in your life. It is possible to find a relaxation through a variety of options, not just food.

Clean the cabinets

Clean out your kitchen and dispose of any items that could lead you to indulge in another addiction. Avoid sweets and junk food from your home. Find healthier alternatives that won't get you into trouble next time you are craving something and want to satisfy your cravings. Store bags of vegetables in your fridge which have been cut for snacks. Make sure you have plenty of fruits. Keep a container of ice-cold water at hand and sip a tall beverage whenever you think about spending money on snacks. It will allow you to be full and stay in the right direction.

Learn About Portion Control

Limit your portion sizes to avoid a crash of calories throughout the day. A quick trick is to use a saucer for every meal. Make sure you only eat what fits onto the table. Try eating small portions of meals throughout the day, instead of taking three larger meals. Make sure to eat healthy meals every couple of hours to help keep your hunger under control and boost your metabolism.

Receive support from others

Keep in mind that there are people who share the same experience. If you join an organization for support, get involved in a chatroom online or form your own circle of friends that share an objective You can always find people who can help you avoid the temptation to eat more. You should have someone you can contact in the event that you're about go to the point of giving in. It's always beneficial to have a steady companion or mentor to help you when you're ready on a food frenzy.

Stay busy

The last thing you want is too much time to relax. Explore and engage in activities during your free time. Don't give yourself the chance to contemplate food. Explore the outdoors, take an excursion for a day or take on an exciting new activity. Don't let grass get in your way and you'll have no time for food comas anymore.

Sometimes, one of the most effective ways to conquer an addiction or disorder is to act. You should try to implement at least any of these methods within the next two weeks , and observe how it will alter your life. Next, try incorporating another approach until you've made progress toward healing and positive changes in your life.

Chapter 10: C-C-E-P Method To Re-Design Your Life

The A-C-C-E-P-T Method is a thought-restructuring system designed to enable you think positively and decision-make appropriately. When you've begun the process of clearing the dust of old patterns of thinking You may be feeling the desire to "redesign" your life. Imagine it as this you're in the right place to revamp your thoughts, just as you'd like to change the look of an old house a fresh appearance. Utilizing the acronym A-C-C E-P-T as an example that you can re-create your personal life

A Accept. As long as we're not able to admit that we're struggling and acknowledge the fact that we need help and help, we're trapped in denial. Instead of being in a state of denial, seek the help that is your Inner Self to provide guidance and strength. Some refer to this universal and spiritual strength "God." Other people consider it to be their conscience. Some people aren't able to relate to those notions, but they know there's a part of them that believes they are able to overcome. One of my clients calls it his "Wise

Self." According to me that it doesn't matter what title you give it. Just call it when you need, and remain attentive as well as open for its divine directions and advice.

The best way to end addiction is to allow people into the habit. While I love to invite your family members or friends to join to join your group The most common issue I encounter when dealing with addictions is that patients are reluctant to tell their story to anyone outside of their comfort zone. This is a serious issue as we do not always follow the advice of our family and acquaintances because they're "too intimate." In addition, we believe (or believe) that they'll continue being there for us despite our flaws. We are relying on our comfort zones that have brought us to the stage of addiction in beginning, and so remaining within them isn't going help us get over them. This is where the community is crucial.

C - Create your life. The most powerful words ever spoken to me were: "You are the creator of your own life. You are the creator of your life." The beginning in my journey was trying to please others and conform to the image I was told to be. What do you think?

I wasn't able to get anywhere and didn't produce very much, and certainly was not very content with who other people said I should be. To be truly content, you have to be completely you. After you've mastered all expectations regarding what others would like from you, and put them aside, you're now in a unique position to begin living, truly living.

Expecting society, your heritage or your parents, your company , your boss, your family , or your spouse to fulfill the purpose of your life and destiny is to not believe that you are in control. There's a chance that you do not believe you're able to start your life fresh. It's possible that you don't feel like you're capable of rebuilding and creating something amazing and extraordinary. But , you are aware that feelings do not always reveal the whole truth. If you've read this book, you've made a significant step towards the right direction. you're becoming more aware each and every day. There is a psychological term that is known as the "Internal Locatus of Control." It refers to those who realize they have the ability to influence the outcomes in their life is their own and not external. There are also people with the "External Locus of Control." These are people who feel a victim and in control. They believe that life is not a matter of chance or it's environmental. Studies have proven that people who have an Internal Locus of Control are much happier and healthier than those who view themselves as victims of circumstances. The different between these two views is that those who have internalized guidance are active people. They don't expect someone else to give them a direction on how to follow. They are ready to make calculated risk and pursue their goals, even if they're not certain what will happen. They trust that when they reach the next fork on the road, they'll be able to determine which direction to take. There is no better way to describe this situation as saying that these people believe in their own abilities. They believe in their abilities to make choices.

Here's a non-clinical definition of intelligence that is appealing my interest "Intelligence refers to the capability to be able to react well to changes." The most intelligent people don't fear change, rather, they make use of it. They don't put on the fence or play the game. They know what's coming and are prepared for it. They say to themselves "I didn't think I'd ever be here however now I'm here. What can I do to get the most out of this circumstance?" That is an intelligent bird. If we allow the thoughts that are automatic and addictive that we accept defeat, we're accepting defeat. We go down without fighting, this is the reason why those suffering from addictions have issues with their self-esteem. Some clients inform me that they have a part of them that constantly tells they are not alone, and insisting to conquer the habit, but an additional part thinks they're locked in a shackle that is unbreakable. In the realm of psychology it's known as polarity in personality. Every person isn't suffering from compulsive or addictive behavior However, I am confident that there are two opposing views. Gestalt Therapy is founded on this notion that we all struggle internally trying to "doing what is right." Hollywood has depicted this inner polarity as a devil standing on one shoulder, and an angel on the other shoulder and both whispering in your the ear. To create your ideal life, you need to be ready and determined to determine the direction of your fate.

Life was never meant to be perfect. If you're prone to an obsession with perfection, I'll remind you that It's messy. In relationships, or on working, there are mistakes because it's part the human condition. Consider the ways a child learns through its mistakes! You learned to not be near fire after putting your finger on something hot. Humans learn how to behave by first learning what they shouldn't do. When you are on the road to recovery, when you slip up and then relapse back to your addiction, don't hesitate to be a bit guilty for a while before letting it go. Then, you can get over it. My experience has been that it's the patients who remain ensconced in shame and guilt that return to the addiction. This means they quit trying and quit in the wake of a single slip up. Remember: A lapse isn't an opportunity to repeated relapse. It's only when you give up on. I heard a wise pastor tell me once, "Never stop starting." If you experience an error, you should remind yourself, "It's part of the process of recovery. I'm not failing when I begin over. I'll simply start from scratch."

T - Thank-Giving. Every one of us has something to be thankful for. Many of us are healthy while others have the riches of others, while others have families Some have friends, others have satisfying jobs, while others have comforting and loving pets, others are devoted to God...whatever you're thankful for, you should celebrate your accomplishments. This is Oprah Winfrey who said, "You can have everything but you can't do everything in one go." Perhaps one day you'll have it all and I'm sure you will. However, until then start your daily routine to work on appreciating the small things you have. Recognizing the little things that are working for us (even even if it's something as basic as a tasty cup of coffee) helps us realize that things aren't always bad. If we can practice the power of gratitude, our lives seem to have an unbiased and realistic viewpoint. If you establish an habit to appreciate the best moments that you experience, then your mood will change, and you will be more enthused by your company. In the end, a person who is grateful is a cheerful person.

Self-Intervention Exercises:

A-C-C-E-P-T

1. Accept More Perspective

Write down what you believe your higher Self or your Wise-Self might have to say to your today about your healing:

2. Building Community

Write a paragraph that describes the ideal community support for recovery could be for you and the reasons for it:

Write a short statement about what you do not want to see in the community support program and the reason for this:

Create a written statement that outlines the actions you can do to gain support from the community:

It is possible to (list the actions):

3. Make Your Life

A. What are you working on today that could be the most beneficial to your life? (Coping techniques and medical intervention, communicating in relationships, etc.):

B. To make your life optimal, what are few things that need to be distinct?

C. What would you do right now, if you knew that you could not fail?

4. Everyone stumbles

If you are experiencing an lapse, what's your plan of action? (Removing Triggers, Urge Surf, Emergency Coping List, Chair Exercise/Reparenting, etc.)

A. Assess your ability to seek out support during an elapse (0-10 zero=will not and 10 = certain Will):

B. What are some proactive actions you can be taking to ensure you don't get trigger-happy?

5. Positive

A. What do you want to happen and what would be your hopes? What's the most logical next step to take in your development?

B. What post-traumatic changes do you recognize that took place in your life because of your situation? (Example: "My problem has made me realize that I need to ...")

C. What specific self-intervention techniques are you doing to enhance your post-traumatic recovery? (Positive affirmations exercise for body awareness and mind-awareness exercises)

6. Thanks-Giving

A. What strengths do I have?

B. What assets do you have in your surroundings that could aid you in reaching your goals for recovery?

C. Who would you like to honor for their contribution to your life? Please list them below, and tell us how they've helped you

Include any additional thoughts you have regarding your experience here:

Chapter 11: The Body Says It Wants!

In the tenth principle, as a continuation of the 10th principle, we can see that by deciding to split foods between "good" as well as "bad," we create an unnatural, deformed food industry in ourselves. The concept of "tasty" that is made of fresh and natural ingredients pleasant, providing sensual pleasure will shift to the notion of "harmful" and "forbidden," so when they attempt to market products for us to call it "tasty," they'll necessarily include something that according to the maker represents the desire of chocolate, icing as well as fat-based cream.

The food you eat should be delicious nutritious, pleasant, and satisfying. It is important to remember that "goodies" aren't all-encompassing - what your body is craving today is delicious. If you're looking for an ice cream cake and you decide to spread sugar-free jam on crackers then you finish eating a cracker packet and an entire jar of jam. If you when you overeat, you're feeling bad emotionally and physically however, the "taste desire" will not go away. you'll want marzipan cake. It will definitely "lie waiting" for

138

you, whether it's at a party with friends at a birthday celebration or in a café and even at a retail store for discounts at the check-out and you'll not have to worry about it as, instead of just eating a single piece consume it's all yours, in vain or some other thing, for which you've endured and was afflicted with. It doesn't say that you are in control. the power of unmet needs as an "salmon" will cause you to swim downstream to spawn, if you consume a marzipan cake at a moment when you're craving it. Voila! It's solved. The requirement is met Then it slumbers and calmly closes itself up for the next time and then disaster doesn't happen.

Training: "How I Make Food Decisions"

1.) Examine and make an outline of what you do to make your decisions regarding nutrition which is primarily based on the food you consume. Examples:

a. Consume what's in the refrigerator

B. Eat what you have left from yesterday or the food that is threatening to get worse;

C. I purchase food at the cafe or cook food in the dining area which is more affordable;

D. I look at what my friends take in and make the same choices.

2.) Keep in mind the largest number of scenarios and attempt to explain all possible alternatives. If you've had a lot of time of experience with diets, you're likely to have plenty of knowledge that you may not want to experience. If you're a follower of strict food guidelines that force you to eat in the most cautious way possible, and to the detriment of your body, then you've also experienced a lot of those experiences. This means it might not be feasible to know what your body requires right away. This is fine. It's just an artifact, and can be learned.

Look at your list. Are there items that say "Eat what I'm craving at the moment"? No?

3.) Make sure you take your time and carefully cross out all of the items listed on your list. Finally, include this one: "I eat what I would like at the moment." From this point on, you'll strictly eat in this or that in this way.

The Search for Signs of Satisfaction with Food

As of now, we've learned a fundamental ability that is essential to the development of intuitive Nutrition that is the ability to eat and feel a certain, moderate level of hunger. We also attempted to determine the degree of saturation that is created due to eating. Saturation is a physiological condition However, the level of satisfaction that food provides is psychological as well as physiological.

Take note of what you've eaten recently. If you ate your meals according to the principles of optimal combinations and you are satisfied with your food, then you will are likely to have a good level of satisfaction from food. That means that, after eating you're in an emotional state and you can feel how you feel about the food you consume. However, it's not just. You feel comfortable recalling the aroma, color of the food you've just eaten and you're happy to remember the picture of the dish, and the details of this dinner.

141

It's difficult to attain the highest level of satisfaction with food in the event that you returned home hungry the glass was empty. You then hurriedly and in despair of being hungry and hung out at the doorway of the refrigerator, soaked in anger. It is impossible to achieve an incredibly high level of satisfaction eating food, even when you have read, watched a film or viewed your emails while eating. An elevated level of nutritional satisfaction does not require only eating the "right" food, that you are craving today, but also a place that allows you to truly enjoy your food. When you eat with a high degree of satisfaction with nutrition is a quick way to notice that you consume less food you need for satisfaction is less.

It is important to note that levels of satiety and satisfaction can differ. In some instances it is possible to eat to a very high amount of satiety. When you are "full," the glass is nearly full or filled, but the degree of food satisfaction , enjoyment and comfort aren't as high. This can happen if you've eaten fast, in uncomfortable conditions or if you did not eat the food you wanted to take in. The reverse could be the opposite that the saturation level isn't very high, you only ate some, but your glass was half empty, but the pleasure the food gives you is the best.

Look for the Best Combination

How do you decide what you're craving in the present moment? Do not think about it in "terms of foods," but in "terms of quality" hot and sweet crumbly, buttery perhaps buckwheat porridge , with butter and sugar. Cool liquid, sour or sweet like kefir as well as sour soup for summer or perhaps iced tea with lemon?

Chapter 12: Finding Peace With Your God-Given Shape

In the modern world it is widely accepted that the body isn't an enlightened, self-regulating and harmonious system in reality, but an uncontrolled animal that needs to be controlled and treated with utmost sensitivity. The tyranny and sexism of unrealistic body perfection and portrayed in the media.

It is a negative, hostile attitude toward one's body that could be "betrayed" at any moment or not wanting to participate in sports or eat foods that are forbidden that regardless of the effort it is not up to the standards of glossy magazines.

It is the result that is painful experiences of body hatred and body shame that are usually the root of another attempt to follow an exercise program or go to the fitness center. The majority of these efforts will fail which results in even more displeasure and even more hatred. Thus, the shift to a more logical and well-informed diet is not possible without changing the way one views your body. The way to living a healthy life that is free of diets and over-indulgence starts when you

144

can accept your body for its current state. The history of a negative view of the body may turn into a long-running one that making changes requires exertion and may not be easy.

What is the best place to begin the journey towards self-acceptance? Three essential things such as mirrors, cabinets, and scales.

Cabinets

In the story I'm about to tell there are many who can identify their own. A young lady, totally fitting into the psychological characteristics of those who are compulsive eaters is overweight, enjoys shopping and eating. The girl has great sense of taste, and she is familiar with the luxury brands to the point of being a complete expert. In one of her trips to the same locations she finds her Dream Dress. The dress was designed by a Fashion Designer and costs, along together with the discounts and sales on the other items 500 dollars. It's a lot for a woman, but she's just trying to love her own self and not be influenced by something else? Can you pay for it? You can afford it!

It is, of course, two sizes smaller than what is needed and doesn't converge on the abdomen and chest. "After all, I'll never shed pounds!" So from the topic of indulgence, my dear dress turns into an act of punishment and an axe of Damocles that hangs over our heroine, who is always met upon when she opens the wardrobe. "You are my displeasure," says Dress. "You still haven't shed any weight and I'm not able to put me at a dance ... It is likely that I will never get in." Since I need to have earned it."

The girl didn't have to be gorgeous She needed an elusive, beautiful objective that this Dress truly represented. Through psychotherapeutic treatment, she began selling branded items that were too big to herself on the online market. The most important thing was that she was astonished by the fact that the profits from these sales was only a small amount. While she was able to sell things inexpensively, she was hoping to clear the items as fast as she could. "Why did I torture myself like this?" She asked herself with a lot of thought, pondering the issue.

What number of clothes are you hanging from your closet? If you've got been through a lot of battles against your body, then the answer is at minimum three. The first is the size you're currently wearing. The other is clothing for when you improve. The third one is clothes in the event that you lose weight. These are clothes is not something you can wear at present but you are hoping to start wearing in the near in the near future. Many weight loss programs urge clients to wear "slim" clothing - it is believed to motivate participants to stick to a diet plan and to train. Consider what you feel in a cupboard. It will likely be sadness, discontent and discontent. The presence of clothing in a closet you are unable to fit in the space is a cause for alarm and usually leads to the consequence of eating too much.

Imagine opening the closet in which you hang your clothes each day. There are plenty of clothes hanging that you aren't able to fit, because they're not big enough for your needs. Some clothes will fit your body but you don't enjoy it a lot and you're exhausted and there's a lot of black or dark clothing in dark hues. A lot of things don't fit together because you don't make any wardrobe choices, or buy things as you wait to lose weight. You should buy the clothes you truly enjoy.

Imagine opening an outfit closet that are your size. You could put on all of the items. Styles and colors represent your mood, condition. What do you feel when you look at this dresser? What are the effects of these feelings on your mood throughout the day?

Inventory Task

Take a look through the closets that your clothes are hung and take out any that don't fit in terms of size. Create a list of the items left. Make a list of what you're missing in order to make your wardrobe filled, and then fill it with clothes that are the same size as your current. The most common responses to this endeavor is complaints of the scarcity of cash to buy items as well as the inability to find clothes stores that cater to large individuals. This and another issue is a way of expressing resistance and a lack of large clothing is also a factor.

Scales

Scales are medical instruments that were invented to assess the weight of a person. Nowadays, they are now an instrument that aids and increases the feeling of discontent in one's body. People who are obsessed with their weight, give the scales' power to decide if they experience a "good" today or "bad" present. A lot of people weigh themselves numerous times during the day, hoping for the numbers decrease, make sure to use the bathroom specifically or take off jewelry prior to sitting at the counter.

Utilizing the scale to manage your diet is doomed to fail. Many people who notice an increase in weight, display symptoms of stress: more anxiety or panic attacks, a decreased mood, and this greatly increases the chance of eating too much. If the scales show a reduction in weight, that should alleviate the symptoms and provide the necessary support. However, many claim that when the scales display the numbers they want the alarm will only increase and it's a bit scary to not maintain what you've achieved. I'd like to reward myself for finally achieving the result I want, and I feel like "you can eat comfortably now, as everything is fine when you weigh "and that's when I start new phases of food restriction and eating too much.

Additionally, it must be remembered that weights are a poor instrument for determining the size of your body. Muscles are more hefty than fat. When you begin to exercise regularly notice weight gain in the form of weight measurements and their overall fitness and well-being increase. The weight of women varies based on the time of the menstrual cycle and the amount of hormones.

If you are looking to establish an enlightened connection with your physical body then your most effective method to achieve it is to eliminate the kitchen scales and eliminate the need to weigh.

While doing this you'll have an awareness of whether you're adding the weight you are losing or gaining through the sensation of how your clothes sit on your.

The decision to let go of weights is an essential step toward acceptance of yourself. It is a sign of acknowledging that the weights on the scales are not able to be used as a determining factor for the self-esteem level you have. More important is your perception about your work, relationships and your interests. and other interests.

Mirrors

Another crucial stage in the process of self-acceptance includes using mirrors. People who feel embarrassed about their body have a hard time with mirrors, both at home and in public. Mirrors are also used by people to mock themselves with a vengeance. The goal of using the mirror is to be able to see yourself with a peaceful and tolerant face, instead of judging and demeaning. The key to having a positive appearance is via the transshipment aspect of a non-judgemental, neutral approach. Don't attempt to transform your negative remarks into positive ones in a hurry - it will not work.

In this moment it is crucial to take every opportunity to gaze at your reflection. When you look in the mirror, you should just describe what you see without allowing any evaluations that are negative or positive. "The belly is protruding, round, muscles calves and round hips" Imagine that you're explaining yourself to an expert who is studying the body's structural characteristics of white (or black and brown) races. Explore your body, and get familiar with it. This is the foundation for the relationship that follows.

Don't overlook the fact that the perception of the entire figure as ugly is not common in a variety of cultures and societies. In this regard, I can refer an earlier story.

A young Dutchman who was obese and morbidly overweight and a difficult childhood, where he learned the entire lesson precisely and developed exactly the characteristics needed to make up for the difficult circumstance in his family, was a highly well-liked, modest, determined academic achievement superior who understands how to stay out of relationships, but not be intimate efficiently. Being overweight since during his teenage years and having been exposed to everything teens get in our society, he discovered for himself that "but the truth is that he's intelligent." He was educated to the highest standard and eventually became a accomplished lawyer. However, panic attacks stopped him from delivering a brilliant performance in court, but beyond the confines that surrounded the courtrooms the lawyer had impressive results in the field of business. He believes that he is as ugly and utterly ugly. Two attempts to establish relationships with women end in failing because he's not open, unwilling to share his feelings, not able to feel that he is loved. Relationships are damaged.

In search of a partner for whom his distance isn't an issue, he selects an attractive girl from Thailand who does not speak Dutch. Communicating in a language that isn't native to both of them, English is a good choice, as it gives a assurance of security. the young man is not able to leave relationships within the initial three months. Then he realizes that his girlfriend is physically and sexually attractive. To him, this is an unusual mail message. it is impossible to immediately erase the negative perceptions about his appearance and yet he must be convinced by her. The young man goes through a massive shock of culture when the girl replies to the question of what appears attractive physically in him - your completeness. In Thailand she states that an entire (fat) body is considered attractive, beautiful and deserving of respect.

In this tale the young lawyer's faith in his capacity to be smart, not just but also attractive, grew slowly and gradually. This doesn't happen in a different manner. When you do this task, you'll repeatedly become critical of your body. When this happens it is time to stop the mirror workout even if you've just begun the exercise.

As your encounter with the mirror grows, your enjoyment of life will get better. You won't be surprised by how you appear in photos or video A good understanding of your body will assist. Gradually an even and neutral attitude to how you look will take over the negative and sour attitude. This will result in an improvement in self-confidence and self-esteem.

There are many who at this point notice that, even though positive or neutral images of your body can be easy to maintain at home, doing anything beyond it can cause a lot of anxiety, particularly if the weight is deemed to be excessively heavy. The opinions and remarks of others will be a threat to you when you, in the viewpoint of the commonly accepted culture of thinness, you appear like a man who is large. Don't forget that this is a sign of the resentment these people feel about their bodies. Your self-esteem increases and hurts those around you, drawing attention to your body as well as the acute sensation of their inadequacy.

But, you'll likely observe that negative thoughts regarding the body recur through your mind every day and you'll need to be more active in attempting to improve your relationships with your body. Thoughts about the body that are negative tend to be cultivated in the early years of the adolescent or childhood. The random comments of relatives and parents and

155

comparisons with other thinner or more attractive children, competition among siblings in the family, and rivalries between peers to be the most attractive, and also the familiarity with magazine covers - all of this provides the foundation for the development of a continuous flow of negative thoughts about our body.

The thoughts that are triggered by these issues can be psychologically "toxic" and are the cause for the constant level of anxiety, a decrease in mood, and eating "breakdowns," and are responsible for the development of extreme eating disorders like anorexia and bulimia as well as excessive eating disorder.

The issue of being unhappy with the body of one's choice has become more prevalent and important for teenagers aged between 16 and 25 and in USA an exclusive Health and Body-Education Program has been created for students at universities and colleges. One of the initiatives implemented within the Body Education Program was the introduction Fat Talk Free Weeks, which is a time of no "bold conversation." The program was launched in 2008 and is a five-day awareness and body-positive programs are now held each year across the globe. Within five days during the week, you are not allowed to use words such as "I'm overweight!" "Oh, you are amazing! Have you lost pounds?" "I need to embark on a diet plan," "With the weight you've gained you should not put it on." "Does my tummy appear obese?"- It's simply not allowed. While doing so there are seminars and lectures about the negative impact on the "ideal of being thin" are given.

The results of this program after eight weeks was that 53% women who participated were no longer experiencing the overwhelming effect of their weight on their lives. 48 percent of women who before felt "fat" frequently were either able to no longer feel this in a way, or the durations of these experiences were dramatically decreased. Nearly half of participants who stated that their thoughts and feelings regarding the weight and appearance hinder them from studying saw a dramatic improvement by the conclusion this program.

What is this all about? Words can have a far more powerful impact on us than what we are accustomed to thinking. If you are just flirting and hoping for an answer to your partner or girlfriend, ask your friend: "Am I not fat in this dress?" - You are harming yourself.

In the event of indications of an eating disorder eliminating negative thoughts about your body is an essential step that is not followed by the development of a positive and healthy attitude towards eating is destined to fail.

The Assignment for 4-Step Transformation

Write down some negative thoughts about your body that irritate you the most often and bother people the worst. This could be an impression about a particular area of your body ("I dislike my thigh fats") or even the entire appearance of the body in general ("I seem like a disgusting animal"). Pick one to change.

You are able to carry out the procedure yourself, but working in a group , or as a pair is the ideal method for this. If, as you read this guide and you think that you would like to recommend it to someone you know from acquaintances, friends, or colleagues, then this person is a great candidate for the job.

Stage 1 - Apologizing

Speak out your negative thoughts about your body in the mirror or another person in your group or couple (there may be as numerous people as you'd like within the group) as it were you speaking to him and not about yourself. For instance, "I hate your fat legs," "I feel sick from your sagging body."

Then, after a few seconds and then, out loud apologize for what you've did. Pick the words you believe are appropriate to request forgiveness in this situation.

If you completed this part of the exercise on your own take note of your emotions when you completed the first and the second part. If you participated as a group or in a couple and you have a partner, ask your partner who

159

participated in the exercise to share with the way he felt when you spoke up and when you apologized and then discuss your thoughts.

Stage 2 Confrontation

Ask yourselfwhy you believe that thin hips are superior to full hips? What was the source of this notion to you in the first place when it first popped into your mind? Who said that this is the case and not in any other way? Consider this question each when it pops into your thoughts.

The change in beliefs you hold about yourself doesn't occur on the same day, but asking inquiries to yourself about this subject can are able to "undermine the credibility of their arguments."

Stage 3 Stop

The decision to be positive or not have negative thoughts about your body inside your mind is a the individual's decision. If you do then you permit them to manifest. The negative thoughts about your body is able to be reversed, and the image that you have of your body is able to be altered to a better one. While it isn't an easy task for everyone, the end result is well worth the effort.

Visualization Exercise

Lay down or sit and find a suitable position for your body. Close your eyes and think about any recent negative thoughts about your body that awoke you. Imagine how this thought appears on your computer screen, like it's being printed. Hit"Delete!" Then, we will print an affirmative (or neutral) assertion that doesn't make you feel less valued or hurtful like: "I am saddened by my hips' appearance today, but we're trying to change the issue." When you are trying to find a positive or neutral expression isn't easy Continue to think about your alternatives until you come up with a solution that you select is perfect for you.

Stage 4 - Coding

The final phase of dealing to overcome negative thoughts about your body comes from the concept that was already mentioned earlier that concerns about an unsatisfactorily ideal body, or "wrong" weight will always hide more fundamental issues with relationships with others. Look for the meaning concealed behind the experiences such as "I have an awful fat stomach that looks ugly" or "I'm too fat and loose." What is it that you are experiencing that others will think or judge you as "fat," "a man with a large stomach," "wide-hipped"?

Do you think that you're afraid of drawing the attention of others and are therefore hesitant to dress in bright colors or snap photos? Are you worried about being rejected , and therefore avoid intimacy, and weight is a reason not to meet new people? Perhaps you're avoiding the graduate conferences, and defending your reasons in terms of "loss of form" but you're actually concerned that everyone will be able to see the way in which your former excel student and medalist didn't become someone else than the mother of three children instead of having a successful and successful career? Get this spiraling thought back (you are able to do it by writing it down).

Which is your most common negative impression of the body that pops into your thoughts when you look at your reflection or go out to a gathering or even take a job interview?

1. I am too fat; I look disgusting.

What is it that makes you appear disgusting? What consequences could it bring in the event that you choose to go out?

2. I am not allowed to dress elegantly. I am not allowed to wear red dresses.

What happens if you wearing a dress in red when you leave the home?

3. Everyone will stare at me, so pay attention.

What will it mean to you?

4. It's a nightmare.

The idea that "I am overweight" conceals the fact that attracting the eye of others can be a snore and creates feelings of anxiety. What happens if you shed some weight? It will not disappear, but it will remain there because it's not tied to weight. The weight is just a covering.

Your negative thoughts about your body, and not only about the body , they convey a significant secret message about the problems that are really troubling you and greatly influence your life and actions. The process of confronting these issues is never easy however, it is essential to improve your quality of your life.

Chapter 13: Intuitive Eating And Weight Loss

It's time to start a new year and you're ready to let go of the diet culture. Farewell to dieting, hi Intuitive Eating! You're gaining more intuitive eating guidelines by allowing yourself to eat and watching your appetite and overall. You're gaining ground. You're on the right track! What is the next step when you have to master intuitive eating and wish to improve your fitness levels?

What happens when you and your friends and coworkers are talking about the latest diets, preparing to lose the last 5 pounds? It's possible to feel as if you're on the same side of intuitive eating and simultaneously, you are surrounded by diet-related culture. In the first place, and of primary importance, I have to be able to accept the weight reduction desires. They are sincere and supported by a population that is filled with weight-consciousness and fat-fear. It is likely that you are a longing. If you are faced with the question, "How might I practise mindful eating while still losing pounds?" This book is perfect for you!

I'd like to clarify that the BMI highlights alongside "Stout" aren't necessary and do not belong in the medical vocabulary. The word "fat" is a fetishized word, and BMI does not relate to illness or other unfortunate ailments. Slimness and weight loss aren't indicators of well-being. If you're trying to be an intelligent eater, but in addition, you want to be slimmer then my question to you is: What is the root of the issue? What is the motivation to be more fit coming from? What would you expect to be the outcome in the event that you gain weight? Do you think you will be treated differently? Then recognized and praised? Good and solid? Are you finally ready to put on that swimsuit that you picked up that you wore in secondary school?

Whatever the reason I'd like you to consider how you could be able to accept that your weight at the set point might not be the ideal weight. This can be a stressful experience and I often find that lamenting is beneficial and important. The loss of the body you desire isn't easy, so try to maintain compassion and beauty while you go through this. Are you able to select actions that will influence your health rather than limiting the size of your body? We have learned from research the fact that weight isn't the only thing that causes constant health or wellness issues.

It is becoming increasingly important to focus on our practices and our relationships with food and development, stress family, rest, friends and more. Perhaps weight loss is the result of changes in habits? Indeed. If you want to pursue wellness it is not possible to achieve the same after weight loss. Doing so will cause you to move further from the body's signals and may disrupt the overall flow of fully grasping the your body's intuitive eating.

If you try to control your intuitive eating habits to get slimmer, this is the definition of a diet. By eating intuitively you could get healthy, lose pounds or maintain your weight. These results are acceptable because instead of choosing micromanagement, you're deciding on the possibility of attunement and opportunity. It could also require an commitment from your body in order to believe that it is at its normal setting level. By recognizing your cravings and wholeness, you are giving yourself a complete and unrestricted permission to eat, feeling content in your eating habits, and removing the deep quality and judgment of food, gaining insight into the process that you like and makes you feel better. These are great ways to learn about the intuitive way of eating.

Intuitive eating isn't an efficient solution. It's not a way to "Win" nor "Tumble away from the trend." It's a continuous development process that will alter when you grow older and go through different phases of your life. Variations in weight are common and could be a sign you are thinking about your body and protecting that you.

The process of building trust in your body and acknowledgment could be a lengthy and winding path. The idea of adoring your body can seem impossible but it is actually quite common and significant. Are you able to start by embracing your body? It might be the case that it helps you make the transition to acknowledging.

There are many wonderful ways to consider your body, but they don't involve changing your body's shape or controlling your weight. Below are a few of them! Moving towards accepting and possibly loving your work environment can force you to make choices and options that are the best for every person, not only decisions that may affect your weight. Be aware, however that over time, the urge to lose weight may diminish because you are convinced that your body's a part of you , not against you.

How to live a healthy Lifestyle by Practicing Intuitive eating

It may sound basic. However, for those seeking to end the diet roller coaster trying to be able to eat with a sense of intuition can fail once they realize that it's not as simple and as "Intuitive" -in the way it appears. Have you categorized the food you eat as intriguingor not appealing because of your food preferences or due to marking this food item with the labels "Great" or "Terrible" for a long amount of time?

169

This is how you can explore the dark places and obstructions and use intuitive eating to your advantage.

Don't forget the Hunger-Fullness Diet Do not follow it!

Intuitive eating's growing popularity is evident in the revolving stream of information about itin books and on webcasts, websites, and online social networks however it's not all that much of the information is accurate. It's not shocking that the idea of an appetite-fulfilling practice -- having food whenever you're full, and stopping after you're full has taken hold. Many people are comfortable looking at things from a different way that it moves into a state of 'I must perhaps eat when I'm hungry.' When you eat intuitively you must discover how to get through the blurred zone. It is possible that eating when you're hungry isn't a good idea. For instance, eating cake at a party usually isn't about a desire, but sometimes we're forced to eat something before becoming hungry because we don't get the opportunity to eat later.

Rejecting the diet-related mindset is far more significant than stopping completely to eat. It's tied to changing your perceptions and observing and then escaping into the unknown, the beliefs that stem from diet culture. In fact, a lot of people are currently "Dieting" but aren't aware of it, and limiting their food choices to improve their health rather than weight loss.

Get Ready For Any Chaotic Feeling:

The most frequent fear people are faced with when they start to explore intuitional eating, is, on the possibility of allowing themselves to indulge in the past, a forbidden food and they'll never be able to stop. This is a reasonable concern. "At the point that someone thinks they'll never be able to stop eating their favorite food, it's probably because they've been denied it for a lengthy period of time," she said. "On the off chance you are and are extremely hungry, it's anything however difficult to be concerned that you'll never give up eating."

The intense cravings for food sweets, for instance, are likely to over time reduce even though the shifts from a state of confinement to one of possibility will feel noisy and raucous at the beginning. "It deserves a few months, or however long it takes, to get some noise in the event you require an acceptable relationship with food items that date back to be decades away.

A common misconception is the notion that intuitive eating entails eating whatever you want anytime you're in need. In the case of intuitive eating you are able to eat whatever you want at any time you want but that doesn't mean that you will do it. Inspiring, completeness, satisfaction the way food impacts us -- all of these are enormously important, but intuitive eating is also a process of being attentive and a learning experience. Instead of being a single cheat day, eating intuitively is linked to creating and usinginteroceptive mindfulness, which is paying attention to your body's sensations. Interoceptive mindfulness is the ultimate power when you understand your physical needs and you'll have access to a collection of information to guide you. After quite a few months of diets, it can prove to be difficult to re-connect with the body's signal, Harrison said. The explicit permission to consume food is a risky way to get back into the body's signals.

Disconnect Nutrition From Dieting:

One of the principles of intuitive eating is to ensure your health by eating a balanced diet. But, once people start training for intuition-based eating habits, they frequently claim that they're treating the food badly or they worry that "Diet mentality" is slipping back in when they're in need of broccoli, salmon and Quinoa instead of fries and cheeseburgers.

People who are intuitive don't feel guilty about eating doughnuts or a bowl of mixed greens, but the confusion is understandable. It is important to ask yourself what's the reason that drives the urge to eat food that is solid? If the intention is to tighten your body, then this is a signal that the psyche of your diet influences every aspect of your life.

There are a variety of clues that point to the looming of blame or fear. In the event that there's any resentment that says, "If I don't eat this broccoli, I'm likely be ill or gain pounds,' these are indications that the diet thinking is creeping into. She points out that choosing broccoli can be an act of self-care. Maybe you've noticed that when you add some portions of vegetables into your diet you're more energetic and your processing is improved. An authentically quiet relationship in the kitchen is about personal care not a matter of discretion.

Allow Time for Intuitive Eating To Feel Intuitive:

While there are ten intuitive eating guidelines, they're not absolute guidelines. There's no such thing that isn't passable or fall short. There is discovering and experimenting. In this regard it is likely that you had a supper to die for. It is important to understand what happens. Maybe you don't feel hungry enough to eat a meal at the end of the day or perhaps you're not as hungry for supper. In the end, it's not satisfying eating less than you should, and it's usually not the best choice to eat too much but you have the option of choosing."

It's generally easy to eat beginning because there's an a plan to follow and clearly defined guidelines. However it is more diligent over time, as the guidelines aren't sustainable and our bodies tend to resist the growing limit. The opposite of intuitive eating is it's hard at the beginning because for lots of people, it's a lot more complicated in comparison to what they've previously done however after a few months intuitive eating becomes easy and unadorned.

Finally, it's linked to returning the enjoyment of food , and also about restoring your relationship with food, brain and body to continue living the best you can in your life.

A Habit of Eating to Break living the Intuitive Lifestyle.

You've stocked your kitchen with nutritious meals and planned carefully-planned meals to get into shape. However it's not functioning. Sound natural? Surprisingly, it could be more than just your storage space which requires an update. You might also need to find a way to end bad eating habits in order to obtain the best results.

Are you unsure where to begin? The first step is to determine those practices that cause damage the most. Check out this list of common eating habits that are void of calories, unfavorable fats or the addition of sugar into your daily diet. Find out which unhealthy habits are familiar. You may not be at all aware that these habits can affect your waistline.

If you identify and focus on the fundamental actions, it becomes simpler to search for answers and observe real results in the form of a scale. If you can identify the activity you want to eliminate then you'll have to take it for better behavior. In general, the best way to alter an eating disorder that is unhealthy is to replace it with a healthier method that is simple and more comfortable. In this way, you'll be able to choose the new way of eating constantly.

Use the suggestions listed below each of your undesirable traits as a starting point for transformation. If you are unsure, alter the suggestions to suit your personal style of living. You could even be creative and design an arrangement that is a good sign for your future.

Recognize The Particular Habit

The main issue you have to tackle is the way you choose to convey your food habits. Just saying "Awful" could be an encouraging step. Making judgments about practices could cause weight loss. The purpose of shame is not to help; experts are prepared to tackle the eating habits they recommend without judgement.

There's no perfect way to eat and nobody is an expert on negative habits. Experts have designed it to help people eat in a way that's healthy and comfortable. So, my clients will surely help them with their diet. Whatever your situation, whether you're using an experienced professional or attempting to alter your habits on your own A moderate and gentle method is the best. Take each habit at a time and set an aim to find simple substitutes that will help you with diet and overall health.

Maintain A Proper Kitchen Decorum:

Once you've let go of the judgement, it's an ideal time to boost your diet by creating a space to make progress. The best place to start is in the kitchen.

Do you store unhealthy food items on the counter of your kitchen? Do you store void calorie nibble foods in eye-level cupboards? Are sugary drinks, scraps or even greasy sweet snacks taking over the middle racks in the cooler? This food stockpiling tendency could cause a surge of unhealthy, uncontrolled eating habits.

Sound Habit Swap:

Place food items that have no calories in areas where you're less likely to be able to view them often.

Keep snacks and chips in the lowest cupboards or up high which means you have to work just a bit to get these items.

Clean your kitchen counters and replace the treat bowl with natural bowls for your products.

Do a full refrigerator overhaul so that when you go into the kitchen to browse the best foods for health are right there.

Keep an eye on your Calories:

If you are a cook who loves to cook then you're already in first place with regards to smart diets or weight loss. When you prepare and plan healthy meals in your home kitchen, it will end into a lot easier to focus on healthy fixings and a bit of control.

However Have you ever ever thought about how many calories you are adding to your daily diet every time you grab the spoon out of the spreader, grab an extra dab of the treat batter or try your homemade pesto mix again and again, and then again? It could mean a lot of calories each day that aren't reflected in your impressive count of calories. In the end, you'll be confused, and possibly abandon the sane diet or weight-loss strategy.

Solid Habit Swap

A water bottle should be kept at your kitchen counter while you cook. When you've used the spatula, spoon or cooking utensil, you can drop it into the water instead of your mouth. It will keep your utensil in good condition and reduce the hidden calories.

Also, make sure you have a sink full of suds ready to soak pots, bowls and other dishes that will entice you. You could also savor an ice-cold mint or bite of sugar gum to deter you from over-tasting while cooking.

Use Distracting Eating as a Method to Practice:

The most effective way to consume more food than you're able to (and increase the weight of you weight) is to try the art of diverted eating. If you tend to snack before your television or computer is a sign that you're an active foodie. If you are eating while reading or browsing magazines could distract you of your meal.

If you are feeling more joyful about your dinner, you're bound to eat slowly and make the most of your meals, and notice signs of hunger and completeness with the aim to eat the ideal amount of food. For this, make sure you have a great time with dinner time.

Solid Habit Swap

Place your table in a place, plate and serve your meals (rather than eating from the crate or plastic container) and turn off the television when you dine.

Set aside the magazines and newspapers and focus on the actual feeling of eating. This type of training, referred to as "Mindful Eating" is the most effective method of maintaining a healthy weight, according to various experts.

Quit Sneaking Food:

Food stealing is a nagging tendency that a lot of her clients might wish to alter. Typically, we have good eating habits when other people are around. As an example, for instance, you might enjoy a healthy diet when your partner is near. But, as it happens that when your partner or spouse is snoring and you are tempted to snack on food items that you normally would avoid. One study has found a link between eating meals alone and the risk of developing metabolic illnesses.

It is possible to consider why you'd like to be out of the shadows of strong tendencies when you're isolated from the rest of the world. There are many people who can indulge in whatever they like while nobody else is looking. If this is the norm for you, your diet program could be too expensive and you may have to alter your diet.

Sound Habit Swap:

You also can be certain that healthy foods are available for you to snack on in case you're hungry.

Make sure that you have good tidbits such as the fresh organic food, the pre-cut vegetables or whole grain saltines or nuts are prepared at the time you're ready to use them.

Conclusion

Issues with eating habits can be an indication of a "signboard" to show that more serious issues in life are concealed. The process of identifying and resolving the inner conflicts that were "stored" within us since the beginning of our lives is a huge and challenging task that can be overcome if you possess the tools to accomplish this such as strength, time and motivation. They will appear when you stop worrying over the possibility of eating the cake or not and what the scales are going to show this afternoon, don't avoid going to the event, as there will be plenty of food that is delicious and you'll be losing your weight or feel that you're not fit enough to look great in this dress, and then you are faced you are irritated and yearning for to eat a bland healthy, yet nutritious meal, fantasizing about completely different meals and feeling apprehensive everywhere because you're so miserable with the basic right to eat whatever you want to eat is not allowed!

In reality, you can eat anything and you'll never be bored be eating anywhere. In the end, food is just an aspect of all the pleasures that exist in the world. Be aware the fact that you are an incredible gift, a loyal and faithful servant, your most reliable companion in all of your endeavours.

The body doesn't refuse and will continue to serve you regardless of the circumstances. Be kind to it. Thank it for its blessings. The satisfaction of living an abundant life in the way they react to their surroundings is what makes someone content. You deserve to be happy - I am sure of that. Thank you in advance , on behalf of the body of my friend as well as my own.